PE~~~~ ~~ ~~
THE OSTEOPOROSIS 'EPIDEMIC'

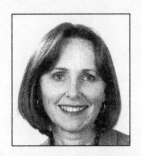

Gill Sanson is a women's health educator and writer. She was Menopause Educator with the New Zealand Family Planning Association Northern Region (1996–2001) and is the author of *Mid-Life Energy and Happiness*, published by Penguin Books (NZ) in 1999. Gill lives in Auckland.

The Osteoporosis 'Epidemic'

Well Women and the Marketing of Fear

Gill Sanson

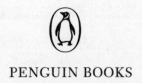

PENGUIN BOOKS

None of the information in this book is intended to be in any way prescriptive or to replace the advice of a physician.

PENGUIN

Penguin Books (NZ) Ltd, cnr Airborne and Rosedale Roads, Albany, Auckland 1310, New Zealand
Penguin Books Ltd, 80 Strand, London WC2R 0RL, England
Penguin USA, 375 Hudson Street, New York, NY 10014,United States
Penguin Books Australia Ltd, 487 Maroondah Highway, Ringwood, Australia 3134
Penguin Books Canada Ltd, 10 Alcorn Avenue, Toronto, Ontario, Canada M4V 3B2
Penguin Books (South Africa) (Pty) Ltd, 24 Sturdee Avenue, Rosebank, Johannesburg 2196, South Africa
Penguin Books India (P) Ltd, 11, Community Centre, Panchsheel Park, New Delhi 110017, India
Penguin Books Ltd, Registered Offices: Harmondsworth, Middlesex, England

First published by Penguin Books (NZ) Ltd, 2001

1 3 5 7 9 10 8 6 4 2

Copyright © Gill Sanson, 2001

Editorial services by Michael Gifkins & Associates
Designed by Mary Egan
Typeset by Egan-Reid Ltd, Auckland
Printed in Australia by McPherson's Printing Group

0 14 100631 5

www.penguin.co.nz
Gill Sanson's website: www.bonestory.com

CONTENTS

For Jude and Camille

ACKNOWLEDGEMENTS

The following people have generously offered invaluable information and resources. They have not been asked to endorse the contents of this book. My grateful thanks to: Dr Susan Ott MD, Associate Professor of Medicine, Washington University who has kindly responded to my every email enquiry; Dr Helen Roberts, FPA research manager and senior lecturer at Auckland University Medical School; Dr Alan Tenenhouse, McGill University Montreal; Dr Max Sutton, Dr Natalia Valentino, Mike Cushman, Cheryl Coleman and the many others who have given support and assistance. A special thanks to the team at the British Columbia Office of Health Technology whose pioneering review of the evidence for bone mineral testing has paved the way for a reconsideration of osteoporosis as it is currently defined, measured and treated. The family is grateful to Dr Tim Cundy in the Endocrinology Department at Auckland Hospital. His research into osteoporosis in young people is where our story really begins.

Grateful thanks to Neil Hamill for his generosity and expertise with legal matters; and to Cordelia Lockett, Anne de Lautour, Dr David Lovell-Smith, Sally Lovell-Smith and Bryan Lee whose opinions and suggestions have been invaluable. Thanks to my daughter Camille for her drawing and graphics, and son Jude and daughter-in-law Mika for help with research. Thanks also to Sandra Coney and Women's Health Action for assistance with illustrations.

Many thanks to Leslie Kenton for encouragement and support in the embryonic stages; and special thanks to Bernice Beachman and Philippa Gerrard of Penguin Books for having confidence in me a second time around, and for their enthusiasm for the project.

Finally, my heartfelt thanks to my wonderful family and my friends, whose constant support is the greatest of blessings. In particular I wish to thank my sister Barbara for allowing me to learn through her experiences, and brother-in-law Ross Johnston for his commitment to getting the story told. My deepest gratitude to Stew who has supported me totally through every stage of this project, and taken care of every aspect of my life during the final push to meet the deadline. It would have been impossible without him.

INTRODUCTION

A family story

IT WAS 1994 AND MY DAUGHTER CAMILLE WAS SIXTEEN. I remember relaxing with visitors when she rang from the fracture clinic at Auckland Hospital. She had been having a follow-up visit for a wrist fracture sustained on the ski slopes a few weeks previously — her sixth. It was the normal sort of teenage call — 'I won't be home for a while, I am going into town to meet some friends.' Then she threw in — 'Oh and by the way, my bones are munted. The doctor who looked at my X-ray says that I have the bones of an 80-year-old.' I was speechless, devastated, and immediately stricken with guilt. I assumed it was something I had done to her — not enough calcium, an inadequate vegetarian diet, some sort of bad mothering for which I would ever pay the price.*

---

* Years later when I consider this event, I am (finally) appalled at the thoughtlessness of the person who told her that. She was young, alone, intimidated, and had no context to place the information in. She tells me now (at age 22) that she immediately cut back on physical activity, *(cont)*

Soon after this we were contacted by the endocrinology department at the hospital and Camille went for a bone densitometry scan which confirmed that she had very low bone mineral density for her age. The relatively recent availability of bone scanning technology had meant that the bone density of young people could be measured for the first time, and it was revealing unexpected variations, prompting a New Zealand study. Extremely low bone density in a young person is a cause for concern because it means he or she hasn't achieved the recognised normal healthy peak bone mass to take them through to adulthood and then older age when bone density naturally declines and fracture risk increases. It was explained to us that existing bone mass is a like a bank credit which can be drawn on. In Camille's case, according to current understanding, she is already in deficit.

Camille had her first fracture at the age of three. She broke her leg when she tripped and fell on the pavement outside our house. Later fractures involved reasonably high-impact falls from a swing and gymnastics equipment, but they were serious. Her elbow was badly broken in one, and both bones in her forearm in another, leaving her permanently unable to pronate (rotate) her left wrist. This effectively terminated any fond notions I had of her becoming a violinist.

A study to determine a genetic risk factor was underway in the endocrinology department at Auckland Hospital and the entire family was invited to participate. Measuring the bone densities of the extended family revealed that my three siblings,

---

(cont) believing her fragile bones could not withstand any knocks or pressure. This, of course, is quite the opposite of what she ought to have done, but no such advice was given. Now she is active, robust and very fit, lifting weights and performing strenuous exercise, which is of great benefit to her bones.

both my parents, my husband, son and daughter, and I all have varying degrees of low bone mineral density (BMD) culminating most seriously in my son and daughter. Six of us have osteoporosis as defined by a BMD of -2.5 standard deviations (SD) below norm or less, and the rest of us have what is called osteopenia, or low bone density, a BMD of -1 SD to -2.5 SDs. Males and females in the family are similarly afflicted, although none of us at this point has fractured since we were children — with the exception of my mother who had a wrist fracture in her 60s.*

Growing up, my sister, brother and I routinely broke wrists, the occasional digit, leg or collarbone, and accepted that this was normal childhood wear-and-tear. In our small town of 14,000 inhabitants, we proudly believed we held the record for the most X-rays at the local hospital. The fracturing eased off as we became adults, and when my children in turn started occasionally breaking their limbs, I stoically assumed the role of fracture-clinic mother, believing this was all a normal part of parenting.

Identifying idiopathic (of unknown origin) osteoporosis in our family raised many questions but no answers. Efforts to determine a cause were inconclusive. Blood DNA samples from individuals in the family and other similarly affected families were sent to Oxford, England, to screen for a common genetic factor. This was unsuccessful in isolating such a gene, although it was clear that there was a genetic link.[1]

For my children it was difficult to know what action to take.

---

* My brother Geoff sustained multiple fractures from a serious tractor accident in 1989. These were not considered to be osteoporosis-related. Any bone will fracture under major impact.

There wasn't any known treatment for very low bone density in a young person. All the tested prescribed treatments were for postmenopausal women with low bone density. Hormonal treatments were inappropriate, and it wasn't clear that non-hormonal treatments would be effective in a young person. Neither was I convinced that the recommended drug (a bisphosphonate) would be safe — given the current lack of data on its use in young people.

Some of us had high levels of the antibodies in our blood which could indicate gluten intolerance or celiac disease. Celiac disease is known to be a 'secondary' risk factor for osteoporosis, as it causes the villi (finger-like projections) in the wall of the small bowel to atrophy or disappear, thereby limiting the absorption of essential minerals. It is believed that maybe one in 300 people have this condition, often without realising it — particularly those of Celtic ethnic origin. The four of us in my immediate family embarked on an 18-month gluten-free diet in the hope that this was the solution. It felt remarkably good to cut out wheat — we all had more energy and better digestion. But disappointingly, after all that time our bone density remained unchanged.

I began to look deeper into possible causes of osteoporosis, ever conscious that the years when peak bone mass is established in a young person (up to about age 20) were almost over for my children. Camille's situation was identified as more serious than her brother's; even though his bone mass was low, hers was significantly lower. A female can be more at risk for additional bone loss during pregnancy, and may lose bone more rapidly after menopause.

This book is the result of my search for an answer for all the members of my family who have this diagnosis. My oldest sister

Barbara, now postmenopausal, was also experiencing increased loss of bone density in her spine and finding herself in the difficult position of having to make treatment decisions on the basis of little information. When the only available information is from drug company pamphlets, it is hard to make a reasoned decision.

But I have a more general interest as well. As an educator of women at menopause, I became inspired to provide information for the vast legions of fearful women who are frequently told that on the grounds of being female, Caucasian and menopausal, that they are very likely to suffer an osteoporotic fracture — perhaps of the spine, probably of the hip, possibly fatally, unless they take long-term and often dangerous medication.

It didn't take long for me to realise that controversy rages over osteoporosis in the higher echelons of the medical world. A few days, weeks and then months of digging through medical journals revealed that low bone density is not deemed a reliable predictor of future fracture. If the disease is defined as a measure of bone density, far more women will have a positive diagnosis than if they are diagnosed in terms of fragility fracture. And the manufacturers of the DXA machines that determine bone mineral density routinely set the 'normal' level against which our bones are measured higher than that recommended by independent researchers. A high reference standard in the bone densitometry machinery means quite simply that many more people can be diagnosed with the disease. Resulting over-diagnosis leads to over-prescription of potentially dangerous drugs, the requirement of regular repeat testing, and untold profit for the diagnostic companies and the osteoporosis drug manufacturers.

The purpose of this book is to provide new information, reassurance, and practical guidelines regarding osteoporosis for men and women of all ages and ethnicities. It is also for their doctors. It includes in-depth information about the effectiveness and safety (or otherwise) of current medical treatments for osteoporosis, along with nutritional and lifestyle information. It also offers a useful guide for what to do after a diagnosis of osteoporosis. As most of the research and the focus of the osteoporosis fraternity have been on European-American women, they will be the main subjects for discussion. This does not, however, limit the usefulness of the book for any reader. Nor is it a reflection of any cultural or gender bias on my part as the author. It is a presentation of the facts as they are currently available.

Read on to find out what you can do to

- Avoid osteoporosis
- Make sure that you get an accurate diagnosis
- Get the appropriate treatment if you are genuinely at risk.

CHAPTER ONE

The epidemic
– is the emperor wearing clothes?

FIFTY YEARS AGO OSTEOPOROSIS WAS RARE. DOCTORS considered it an uncommon bone disease, not a women's disease, and until twenty years ago most of us had never heard of it. Spontaneous fracturing of hips or compressing of vertebrae resulting in painful curvature of the spine were unusual and confined to the very elderly.

You know a disease has really made it when it gets its own internationally recognised day. Since it became one of the top ten diseases, marked by World Osteoporosis Day each October 20th, osteoporosis seems to be everywhere. Now the osteoporosis foundations of the western world are warning of an epidemic. We are told that one in two western women (and one in three men) will suffer a bone-density related fracture in their lifetime; that 20 percent will die within six months of a hip fracture, and another 50 percent will require long-term nursing care.[1] The slogan of the US osteoporosis prevention campaign in May 2001 was 'Every 20 Seconds,

Osteoporosis Causes a Fracture'.[2]

Facts like these suggest that the disease is more widespread than breast cancer, AIDS, and heart disease rolled together. How did this happen and, more importantly, is it true? Where are all these people? Surely our hospital beds should be full of people with fractures, and most elderly women should have severely curved spines ('dowager's humps').

On top of that, a 50 percent increase in the disease is predicted in the next 15 years. World elderly populations are growing, in line with the global population explosion of the last 50 years. It is estimated that 1.7 million hip fractures were suffered by senior citizens in the world in 1990. That number is expected to increase to 6 million by 2050, *based solely on increasing populations and increased life expectancy, not because of any other factor*. The expanded populations in Asia, Africa and South America are expected to lead to massive increases in the numbers of elderly people. As a consequence, and despite the comparatively very low rates of fracture in these countries, there is an expected shifting of the 'burden of the osteoporosis disease' from the developed to the developing world. According to the World Health Organisation Osteoporosis Task Force, 'some 75% of hip fractures are expected to occur there [Asia, South America and Africa] by the year 2050 . . . [Therefore] . . . It will be necessary to develop and disseminate prevention strategies which can be used in these regions.'[3]

In 1998 the incidence of hip fracture in mainland China was one of the lowest in the world.[4] An article on the International Osteoporosis Foundation website now estimates that some *212 million* fractures will occur annually in China by 2050.[5] Predicting an epidemic in these countries provides unlimited commercial opportunities for the 'osteoporosis-preventing' drug, bone density testing, calcium and dairy industries, which already make unprecedented profits from sales in Europe, the US, Australasia and Japan.

ANN'S STORY

As Ann levered herself off the radiology table after her bone densitometry test, the technician assessing the computerised results warned her that by the time she was 80 she could 'be in big trouble'. Ann felt shocked and very anxious. A follow-up visit to a specialist confirmed that she had 'decreased bone density', and included advice that she should immediately begin a calcium supplement programme, and return for a scan in two years time in order to monitor what was potentially a situation of great concern. Her low bone density was blamed on a life-long aversion to dairy products, and the close proximity of two pregnancies followed by lengthy periods of breastfeeding.

Ann had agreed to have a bone scan at age 45 because her doctor recommended it as a routine and responsible thing to do as she entered the menopause transition. She is a very fit person, of small build, has no family history of osteoporosis, an excellent diet, doesn't smoke, drink, take any medications or have a personal history of low-trauma fractures.

Ann doesn't have osteoporosis, she has osteopenia or low bone density, and even that diagnosis is questionable given the wide variation of measurements with bone density densitometry (DXA) machines.[6] In reality, this level of bone density may well be normal for her, and labelling it 'decreased bone density' as the specialist did is puzzling as there was no way of knowing what Ann's bone density had previously been.

Neither did the test tell her about the *strength* of her bones — it isn't able to do that.

What the specialist could have done was reassure Ann that her bones are probably normal, if on the low side of normal because she is a small person.[7] He could have told her that BMD is only a fraction of the osteoporosis story and that in the absence of other risk factors, her chances of having a fracture as a result of fragile bones are minimal.[8] He could have told her that there is no evidence that dairy foods reduce the risk of fracture, and that her diet was more than adequate.[9] He could have reassured her that even though bone density may be lost during pregnancy and lactation, bone density recovers quickly, even if the intervals between pregnancies are short.[10] He could have encouraged her to remain fit and to do weight-bearing exercise, and to take, if anything, a balanced bone nutrient supplement. Instead he has added her to the ever-growing list of 'worried well' women who believe themselves candidates for a crippling disease.

There is something deeply disquieting about being told that you have osteoporosis, particularly in the absence of symptoms of disease. It is a bit like hearing that your cherished family home is structurally unsound, that termites or borer have eaten away at the foundations and it could collapse at any time. But you do have the choice to move to another building. When it is your body, the effect of a diagnosis can be shattering. People react in different ways. Although very little attention has been paid to the psychological effect of such a diagnosis, one study showed that many women stopped exercising or lifting heavy objects, and generally limited physical activity after being told they were at risk for fracture — the very opposite of what is recommended.[11] Others immediately embark upon long-term drug regimes which may put them at greater risk for more life-threatening conditions than a broken wrist bone, or a loss of height.[12]

Osteoporosis

Osteoporosis is a condition where bones fracture as a result of little impact or trauma because they have become thin, brittle, and have lost tensile strength. Osteoporosis and complications arising from loss of bone mass and strength in the elderly have been present in human populations for thousands of years, but have always been recorded as affecting only a fraction of the population. Although there is little recorded evidence of the disease in antiquity, the skeleton of a postmenopausal woman from Lisht, Upper Egypt, dated to the XIIth Dynasty (1990–1786 BC) has been recently scanned to reveal a hip fracture and compression fractures of some of the vertebrae.[13]

Everybody loses bone density as they age, but the vast majority of the population never fracture as a result of low bone density. Osteoporosis as defined by fragility fractures is uncommon, even rare, in women under the age of 80. It afflicts mainly very elderly people in the form of hip fractures, and a smaller percentage of younger women and men. Fractures are likely to occur in the presence of other factors involving illness and frailty: immobility, dementia, medication such as corticosteroids, anti-depressants and sleeping pills, and malnutrition. Under these conditions, an elderly person may fall and fracture their hip. The older a person is and the more unwell they are, the greater the risk. Other than maintaining a good level of health and fitness, there is nothing a well woman in her 50s and 60s can do that will avert such an event.

Osteoporosis is a serious condition with potentially

devastating consequences for the genuine sufferer. But it is one of the most commercially profitable diseases ever because it targets and 'diagnoses' the worried well — a vast market of supposedly at-risk people who can be convinced to take expensive tests and drugs to prevent something which most of them will probably never have.

Osteoporosis is diagnosed as a disease when, in most cases, it isn't. People are diagnosed with osteoporosis because they have low bone density (BMD) not because they have fractured. This despite the fact that BMD testing does *not* accurately identify women who will go on to fracture as they age.[14] Women with high bone density may fracture, and others with low bone density may fracture too. Low BMD is one of many risk factors for a condition which in the end can only be truly diagnosed when there is a 'fragility' fracture (a fracture as a result of low impact or trauma). Calling low BMD osteoporosis is like calling elevated cholesterol heart disease, or high blood pressure a stroke.

The vast majority of postmenopausal women need not be concerned about osteoporosis. There is substantial evidence that good diet, a healthy lifestyle and regular exercise are sufficient protection against future fracture. Even the experts agree. Mark Helfand, one of the members of the US National Institutes of Health (NIH) consensus panel that spent three days in March 2000 conferring about the prevention, diagnosis and treatment of osteoporosis, had this to say in a recent *Washington Post* article: 'I think even people who agree that osteoporosis is a serious health problem can still say it is being hyped. It is hyped. Most of what you could do to prevent osteoporosis later in life has nothing to do with getting a test or taking a drug.'[15]

Misleading advertising

The information from osteoporosis literature, most doctors, advertising, and the media is misleading, often inaccurate, and has been allowed to proliferate unchecked without public policy and objective analysis. Despite contradictory challenging evidence being published repeatedly in prestigious medical journals, the front-line promoters of the osteoporosis industry present a convincing message that virtually all women over the age of fifty years face the spectre of debilitating pain, loss of independence, and immobility as a result of a crumbling spine or a fractured hip. That is, of course, unless they avail themselves of the technology and the medication that will diagnose, treat and 'cure' them.

For every statement from the medical establishment that you read or hear on the prevalence, diagnosis and treatment of osteoporosis, there are evidence-based articles and reviews which oppose them. This 'other side' of the story is known to the osteoporosis specialists and those who stay informed. It has been published in the medical literature, discussed at consensus conferences, yet has somehow failed to filter through to the public and to doctors who help 'at risk' patients make decisions regarding their bone health. What reaches many general practitioners and their patients are not facts at all, but opinions. So much is not known and, as a consequence, just about every aspect of osteoporosis is a matter of hot debate.

The commercial return is substantial for an industry that has emerged with lightning speed in recent years. The immense profits generated by these companies will increase as more and more of the greying female baby-boom population acquire a 'risk factor' for osteoporosis simply by virtue of their age — reason enough to perpetuate the idea of the seeming inevitability of postmenopausal hip fractures and a subsequent life of disability and dependency.

A recent report predicts that the hormone replacement (HRT) market will grow from $2.7 billion in 1998 to $5.9 billion in 2008 in Europe, the US and Japan alone.[16] All this despite the fact that HRT, which is recognised as the 'gold standard'* treatment for osteoporosis, is increasingly controversial because of serious risks associated with its use, unpleasant side-effects and a lack of benefit. Remarkably, conclusive evidence of its effectiveness in preventing fracture has yet to be determined.

The marketing of fear

In the early 1980s most women had never heard of osteoporosis, and most doctors saw very few patients with the disease. But that was all about to change. In 1982 a major promotional campaign sponsored by the Ayerst pharmaceutical company set about creating public awareness of osteoporosis as an important women's health issue. Ayerst (now Wyeth Ayerst) is the world's biggest producer of hormone replacement therapy in the form of Premarin, the equine oestrogen collected from the urine of pregnant mares.**

The campaign included massive radio, television and magazine coverage with articles and advertisements published in *Vogue*, *McCall's* and *Reader's Digest*. Although the focus of

---

* The term 'gold standard' is used in medicine to identify a treatment or strategy which is recognised as the safest and most effective.

**International animal rights campaigners raise concerns about the mistreatment of the pregnant mares whose urine is collected during the six-month gestation period. Unable to lie down, the animals are forced to stand in stalls for the duration, and are rarely, if ever, exercised. Their foals are taken from them at birth, fattened and slaughtered for the Japanese market and dog food. Premarin remains the mainstay of the US and Japanese HRT markets.

the campaign was on the disfigurement of the dowager's hump and the damage of the disease, rather than the hormone replacement they were selling, the company clearly stood to benefit from increasing public awareness of osteoporosis. Fearful women who went to their doctor to discuss prevention were likely to end up with a prescription for HRT.

So successful was the campaign, quickly joined by the calcium and dairy industries, that by the mid-1980s most European and American women had not only heard of the

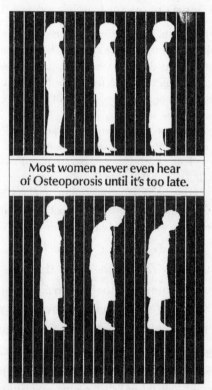

Most women never even hear of Osteoporosis until it's too late.

One of the early advertisements for calcium supplementation. The bent-up old lady became the symbol of the public awareness campaign.

disease, they had accepted and were increasingly fearful of the apparent inevitability of hip fractures and a life of disability and dependency. Women were frightened of becoming like the elderly woman with the severely bent spine in calcium advertisements.[17] The medical profession in turn was convinced that osteoporosis is a crippling disorder that must be identified early and then successfully treated with HRT.

In their review of the evidence for the effectiveness of bone mineral density testing, the British Columbia Office of Health Technology Assessment quotes from a report at the time:

> Many advertisments play on the fear of ageing, such as the spot for a calcium supplement that shows a healthy thirty-year-old woman transformed to a stooped sixty-five-year-old in thirty seconds. While such an image capitalises on the fear of losing youthful beauty, it draws on even deeper fears of disability leading to loss of independence.
>
> The information on hip fractures is equally frightening. For example, a popular guide to preventing osteoporosis states: 'The consequences of osteoporosis can be devastating. Fewer than one-half of all women who suffer a hip fracture regain normal function. Fifteen percent die shortly after their injury, and nearly 30 percent die within a year.' The fear for women is that even if they survive a hip fracture, they may face long years of dependency and immobility.[18]

The advertisements fail to mention that the majority of postmenopausal women who do have spinal (vertebral) fractures are unaware of the fact and have no symptoms, and that most fractures occur only in the very elderly and are linked to many other complicating factors. The truth is that most women who suffer hip fractures are aged 85 or more and are unwell. Many of those who didn't recover would unfortunately have died within a year anyway. While a hip fracture played a part in their deaths, it didn't cause them. It is estimated that as few as 14 percent of deaths following a hip or pelvic fracture were caused or hastened by the fracture in women who were walking and active prior to the event.

The continuing bombardment of advertisements, campaigns in the media and fact sheets in doctors' waiting rooms grossly exaggerates the numbers of people who fracture and the impact that osteoporosis can have on a postmenopausal woman's life.

The re-defining of osteoporosis

In 1994, in the wake of the globally successful osteoporosis marketing campaign, came a new definition of osteoporosis which was so broad that it would catch half the postmenopausal women alive. It would also cement in place the economic futures of the drug and technology manufacturers.

Osteoporosis had previously been characterised by fragility fractures — that is, bones breaking under relatively low impact. If, for example, you fracture your leg in a high-speed skiing accident, or your ribs in a car accident, these are considered *high trauma*, and conditions under which any bone would break. But if you fall off a chair, trip while walking, or stub your toe and a fracture results, these are considered *fragility* fractures.

In 1988 Dual X-ray Absorptiometry (DXA) machinery was developed to measure the bone mineral density (BMD) of an individual as a means to determine the likelihood that person has for developing osteoporosis. DXA has become the internationally recognised gold standard for determining osteoporosis risk. But BMD is measuring only bone mass, not the factors which contribute to bone fragility such as bone size and shape, vertebral body diameter, hip axis length and loss of trabecular cross-bracing.

Bone mineral density naturally decreases with age in all people, but not all people are at risk for fragility fractures. The development of the impressive new and sophisticated DXA technology had reached a point where low BMD was about to be transformed from a risk factor to a disease.

In 1994 a World Health Organisation (WHO) committee of experts established an international standard which now classifies a bone mineral density reading of 2.5 standard deviations (or grades) or more below 'normal' as a diagnosis of *osteoporosis*, and 1 standard deviation to 2.5 standard deviations below 'normal' as a diagnosis of *osteopenia,* or low bone density, the early stage of osteoporosis.* The normal level is currently determined by an assumed average peak bone density of young white women — in most cases, American. This is known as a T-score. For each standard deviation decrease in bone mineral density, doctors are warned that fracture risk in their patient is predicted to double.[19] This means that unless women maintain their bone mass at peak levels throughout their life they will be labelled as at risk or diseased. The natural biological variation among healthy adults, and natural, universal age-related bone loss are not accounted for by this definition. Neither is the all-important fact that low bone density is not a good predictor of fracture risk.

✳ • Normal: a value for bone mineral density or content within 1 standard deviation (SD) of the young adult reference mean.

• Low bone mass (osteopenia): a value for bone mineral density or content more than 1 SD below the young adult mean but less than 2.5 SD below this value.

• Osteoporosis: a value for bone mineral density or content 2.5 SD or more below the young adult mean.

• Severe (established) osteoporosis: a value for bone mineral density or content 2.5 SD or more below the young adult mean in the presence of one or more fragility fractures.

This new definition meant that millions of women suddenly qualified for diagnosis of a disease for which they had never considered themselves at risk. As one expert in osteoporosis recently put it: 'The number of people with "low bone density" depends very much on how you define it. If you want to make more people have osteoporosis, simply change the definition of osteoporosis or use a kind of bone density measurement that decreases with age [i.e. the T-score].'[20]

Both these things have happened. The definition of osteoporosis has changed from fragility fractures to a measure of bone density. The 'normal' level is that of young person with high bone density. That ensures that age-related decrease in bone density is automatically categorised as abnormal.

Powerful market forces

The market forces behind the redefining of osteoporosis are appreciable because once a woman has been diagnosed as having low bone density, she is hooked into a lifetime of screening, monitoring, and potential drug therapy. A massive global industry involving drug and device companies, calcium suppliers, and the dairy industry has emerged and grown rapidly to support the new 'epidemic'. A recent article challenging the validity of the new definition states:[21]

> In the time leading up to the WHO redefinition of osteoporosis, drug companies were poised and waiting, recognising that a massive potential target population of baby boomers existed and was growing. In 1992, only an estimated 15% of the female population in the United States received some form of hormone therapy, making the economic implications of the WHO-sanctioned redefinition quite staggering. . . . [It was] no small inducement for commercial interests to foster a climate of fear and stimulate the demand for health technologies, whether or not they will lead to measurably improved outcomes.

By 1999 some 37 percent (16 million) of US postmenopausal women were using HRT.[22] The numbers continue to increase despite widespread discrediting of HRT. With 36 million baby boomers now reaching menopause in the US alone, the potential for further sales is enormous.

One assumes that the World Health Organisation is an independent and neutral body, untainted by any conflict of interest in its assessments and reports. But the meeting of the WHO study group on bone densitometry screening which defined the thresholds for diagnosing osteoporosis was funded by three major drug companies which stood to gain from the new definition. They were Rorer Foundation, Sandoz Pharmaceuticals (now called Novartis, the company which produces Calcitonin, a treatment for osteoporosis), and Smith Kline Beecham (now GlaxoSmithKline), the makers of Tums and Oscal calcium products.[23] From this initial meeting emerged similarly funded conferences worldwide, and despite widespread criticism the WHO definition has been adopted as the mainstream measure for diagnosing osteoporosis.

Today many international independent review groups do not sanction the WHO definition, and many have argued against its use. The Swedish Council on Technology Assessment in Health Care (SBU) demonstrated that the WHO's use of healthy young women as a reference group in the definition resulted in large numbers of women being wrongly defined as abnormal. Using these standards, they estimate that 22 percent of all women over the age of 50 will be defined as having osteo-porosis, and 52 percent as having osteopenia. The SBU also raised concerns that 'defining a complex, often lifelong, process such as osteoporosis in terms of a single BMD measurement is highly problematic and should be critically examined'.[24]

Despite concerns, the definition has been widely accepted by the scientific community. The flaws in such a simple definition are many:

1. It concludes that bone density predicts a person's future risk of fracture. It has not been shown conclusively that it can.

2. It assumes that the young reference normal peak bone mass used in the DXA machines is an accurate representation of everyone's peak bone mass gained in early adulthood. As it turns out, peak bone mass is virtually indefinable as it varies from race to race, between genders, seasons, and even geographical regions of a country. Interviewed by a journalist in 1998, Alan Tenenhouse, the principal investigator of a recently published large groundbreaking Canadian study, had this to say: 'The most interesting thing we've learned is that peak bone mass varies across the country . . . We can't find any real differences to explain it. It's substantial. The difference is greater than 10 percent, which is more than one DXA standard deviation.'[25]

3. Most alarmingly, there is no international normal reference standard for DXA machines. Manufacturers set their own, often high standards, resulting in widely varying outcomes and diagnoses across machines, towns, and countries.

4. The criteria really only apply to Caucasian women. It is known that there is a huge variation in bone mass among ethnic groups, and between men and women. A study of four ethnic groupings — Hawaiian, Filipino, Japanese and white women — found differences in peak bone mass of up to 100 percent among the four ethnic groups.[26] It is essential therefore that local population reference standards of the

same ethnicity be used when measuring bone density — something that is rarely done.

The WHO definition was apparently designed to convince the sceptical policymakers at the time of the perceived 'magnitude' of the osteoporosis problem.[27] It was clearly successful in that regard because it has since netted far more of the population than was ever anticipated (or predicted by the standard definition model). Surely this is cause to question such an arbitrary definition? But the osteoporosis societies of the United States and other western countries now routinely state that at least 50 percent of all women over the age of 50 years have osteoporosis (as defined by low bone density).

DXA manufacturers are allied with the drug companies

If low bone density is a disease, then once identified it can be treated with pharmaceuticals. In 1995, hard on the heels of the establishment of the new WHO definition of osteoporosis, Hologic and Lunar, the two biggest international suppliers of bone densitometry machines, formed an alliance with the US drug manufacturer Merck to 'further secure the interests of these two major branches of the industry'. Merck is the company that produces the osteoporosis drug Fosamax (Alendronate), and more recently HRT after the purchase of a Monaco-based HRT manufacturer. Merck subsidises the sale of Hologic and Lunar's DXA machines — particularly to reach areas which were previously unable to afford them, the smaller hospitals or medical practices that had been resisting the expensive technology. A worldwide proliferation of densitometry machines has secured further sales of the pharmaceuticals associated with a diagnosis. In an article published at the time to announce the deal, the intention is clear: 'The trend toward disease management is forging alliances between device manufacturers and pharmaceutical houses that may ultimately benefit both the patient and the corporate bottom line.'[28] The deal has clearly benefited Merck. In 1999 sales of Fosamax rose to $US1 billion worldwide, and in 2000 to $US1.3 billion.

What about fracture rates?

All this is ignoring one essential factor — the presence or otherwise of fracture. Because osteoporosis is all about breaking bones, the preoccupation with measuring bone mineral density tends to eclipse this obvious important indicator. The fact is that you may have low bone density and never fracture. Or you may have normal bone density and fracture. Although it is repeatedly overlooked in the publicised WHO definition of osteoporosis, 'established' osteoporosis is defined by low BMD *along with one or more fractures resulting from low impact or trauma.*

When determining the incidence of osteoporosis, low bone density is not being distinguished from established osteoporosis which is defined by the prevalence of fractures. This creates enormous confusion when trying to make sense of osteoporosis statistics, because in most cases they are based on BMD alone, not fracture rates.

The bone mineral density (BMD) definition of osteoporosis has contributed to the medicalisation of normally ageing women, and supports the use of technology in determining disease. It has resulted in the unchecked proliferation and use of bone densitometry machines in the western world.

All this without evidence for its effectiveness. A Canadian government-funded report on six large international reviews of the evidence for the effectiveness of BMD testing recently concluded: 'BMD testing is unable to accurately distinguish women at low risk of fracture from those at high risk.'[29]

What is the actual risk of fracturing?

Depending on your country of residence, where you seek information, how the disease is defined, and how fracture data is interpreted and presented, a Caucasian woman's estimated likelihood of an osteoporosis-related fracture after the age of 50 years ranges from 10 percent to 56 percent. Most estimates are around the 50 percent range, but fail to explain that this is based on:

- Wrist (or Colles') fractures which tend to happen to women in their 60s and 70s, and may or may not be linked to osteoporosis. There is little evidence that BMD plays a part in these fractures, as DXA measurement of the forearm does not seem to be able to predict them. A Colles' fracture can occur with normal, high, or low bone density of the forearm.[30]

- A loose and hotly debated definition of vertebral 'fractures'. There is really no comparison between the seriousness of hip fractures and vertebral fractures. Most vertebral fractures take the form simply of a loss of height without any major symptoms. According to Dr Bruce Ettinger, an endocrinologist and Clinical Professor of Medicine and Radiology at the University of California: 'Only 5 percent to 7 percent of 70-year-olds will show vertebral collapse; only half of these will have two involved vertebrae; and perhaps one-fifth or one-sixth will have symptoms. I have a very big practice and I have very few bent over patients. There's been a tremendous hullabaloo lately, and there are a lot of worried women — and excessive testing and administration of medications.'[31]

- A 50-year-old woman has a 15 percent chance of a hip fracture by the time she is 80. Hip fractures which occur between the age of 80 and 90 are invariably linked to factors other than osteoporosis. Many elderly people suffer from poor eyesight and other serious medical problems like dementia. Many in this age-group are taking several different drugs including corticosteroids and powerful long-acting tranquillisers or antipsychotics (often simultaneously) that can trigger falls. Falling and breaking a hip therefore is most often a marker of generally frail health, and in most cases has little to do with osteoporosis.[32] In fact, falling in a particular way will fracture the neck of the femur regardless of bone strength or density. A man or woman who remains fit and well is less likely to fracture.

When these factors are taken into account, it is clear that the risk of an osteoporosis-related fracture is nothing like 50 percent. Dr Bruce Ettinger reassures further: 'Women shouldn't worry about osteoporosis. The osteoporosis that causes pain and disability is a very rare disease.'[33]

Despite this, advertising campaigns in the media, and literature circulated in doctors' waiting rooms and pharmacies, warn women in their forties, fifties and sixties that they must take action now to avert a life-threatening disease which can bring death, disability, deformity and loss of independence. Vulnerable women and men are easy targets for the persuasive marketing strategies of the drug companies, the medical profession and the calcium and dairy industries.

In the absence of internationally agreed criteria for measuring fracture statistics and because of the confusion over the BMD definition, the following statements indicate the widely diverging 'absolutes' in the osteoporosis message:

- *Osteoporosis New Zealand*: Osteoporosis is a major health issue with 56 percent of all postmenopausal women predicted to have an osteoporosis-related fracture.*[34]

- The *Mayo Clinic*: In the USA, about 21 percent of postmenopausal women have osteoporosis and about 16 percent have had a fracture.[35]

- *US National Osteoporosis Foundation*: One in two women and one in eight men over age 50 will have an osteoporosis-related fracture in their lifetime.[36]

- The *Canadian Multi-Centered Osteoporosis Study (2000)*: In Canada approximately 16 percent of women and five percent of men suffer from osteoporosis.[37]

---

* New Zealand's alarming prediction is based on a 1994 Australian epidemiological study. A close look at the study reveals that it involved the analysis of 271 low-trauma fractures sustained from 1989 to 1992 among 2000 women and 1508 men aged 60 years or more in the town of Dubbo in New South Wales. Believing Dubbo to be a population representative of elderly Australians in terms of recognised fracture risks such as tobacco and alcohol usage, prescribed medication, weight, height and overall health status, the researchers extrapolated from the results what the fracture statistics of the whole Australian population for that period would have been. Thus 58 hip fractures, 15 vertebral fractures, and 57 forearm fractures, among others, were multiplied to become a national total of 72,520. As a consequence and after further calculations, Australian women are warned that they have a 56 percent likelihood of a fracture after the age of 60 years. Men have a 29 percent likelihood. In the absence of a similar local study, Osteoporosis New Zealand promotes the same data in its literature, despite known variations in fracture incidence between countries, and between regions in countries. (*Osteoporosis International* 1994; 4: 277–282.) For example, hip fracture incidence in New Zealand has been found to vary widely from region to region. (*NZ Med J* 1997; 110: 78–80.)

- *National Health and Nutrition Examination Survey III*: The age-adjusted prevalence of osteoporosis in women aged 50 years and older was 21 percent in US whites, compared to 16 percent for Mexican Americans and 10 percent for African Americans.[38]

- *International Osteoporosis Foundation*: Worldwide, the lifetime risk for a woman to have an osteoporotic fracture is 30–40 percent. In men the risk is about 13 percent.[39]

- *National Osteoporosis Society UK*: 1 in 3 women and at least 1 in 12 men will develop osteoporosis during their lifetime.[40]

- *Australian Osteoporosis Society*: It is estimated that the proportion of women with osteoporosis increases from 15 percent in those aged 60 to 64 years up to 71 percent in those over 80 years of age. The incidence is much lower in men, ranging from 1.6 percent of those aged 60 to 64 years to 19 percent of those aged over 80 years.[41]

An article appeared in the *NZ Herald* in April 2001, quoting Professor Ian Reid, from the Auckland Medical School, as saying: 'People might be surprised to know that everyone had osteoporosis, though most to a lesser extent. No one is immune to it really. It is a condition we all have after 40.'[42] When osteoporosis is defined only in terms of a measure of bone density and when the normal reference standard is that of a young person, it is almost inevitable that everyone has it after age forty. Without information on the incidence of fragility fractures, however, it is a meaningless definition.

Difficulties in determining fracture statistics

Statements on the incidence of fracture are constructed from data that is open to wide interpretation. Dr Susan Ott, an

international osteoporosis authority from Washington
University, comments:

> Counting the actual number of fractures related to osteoporosis is
> more difficult than it appears and requires strict criteria. It would
> be quite easy to make the figures high if you wanted. Obviously a
> huge number of people fracture as the result of accidents, and who
> says how many of those should be counted? What actually
> constitutes a fracture of spinal vertebrae is also dependent upon
> how the vertebrae are measured. Loss of height has been used as a
> measure and when a small amount of height loss is applied then
> fracture rates are very high. However, when stricter criteria
> involving spinal X-rays and measurement of vertebrae are involved
> there are far fewer fractures.[43]

And how do you decide? In a recent medical journal article,
osteoporosis expert Dr R. P. Heaney says:

> Any bone will break if pressure is applied in a particular way, so
> falling patterns are also a big factor. Even young normal bone will
> fracture if struck just so; many elderly fragility fractures are of
> precisely this sort.[44]

Times have changed

It is also not possible to make the assumption that women
turning 50 now will have the same rate of fracture as the women
who are currently in the high-risk elderly age group. Those
women who are aged 75–100 now were born between 1901
and 1926. Their peak bone mass was being developed up until
the end of World War II — a period which spanned the Great
Depression and two world wars with the associated poverty,
compromised nutrition and disrupted lifestyles. Who is to say
that the women currently entering menopause are going to
have similar fracture rates to their mothers and grandmothers?
Chances are they will be very different, given dietary and
lifestyle changes, and the control the baby boomers have had

over their reproductive history with the consequent fewer pregnancies and greater number of menstrual periods. It is well known that reproductive hormones influence bone metabolism. Circulating ovarian hormone levels are very different in the woman who is repeatedly pregnant and lactating, from the woman who is not. In addition, the long-term effect of exposure to synthetic hormones in the form of the oral contraceptive pill, HRT, and environmental hormone-mimicking chemicals is unknown.

Women and ageing

Western clinical medicine is heavily influenced by popular notions of women and ageing. Younger women of reproductive age are considered the standard for what is normal and healthy, and ageing women's bodies are often considered in terms of hormone deficiency, a condition that needs to be treated with hormone supplements. HRT is therefore heralded as the panacea for the ageing woman. It is reputed to replace the 'missing' hormones, deal with difficulties associated with menopause, and simultaneously halt age-related bone loss, and by definition, osteoporosis.

Ageing in the west is about losses, not gains. The onset of menopause is equated not just with loss of fertility, but also loss of youth (and by association femininity and sexual desirability), and loss of social status. Ours is not a society that tends to place value on life experience and wisdom, so older women can feel a sense of social redundancy. Added to that is the deep fear of disability and the loss of independence.

Magazine articles and books on menopause tend to emphasise the biological changes that occur, and perpetuate the idea that the ageing female body is in a state of decline.

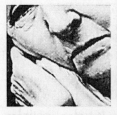 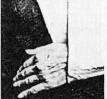 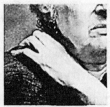
Images such as these of the 'oestrogen deficient' woman dominated early HRT advertising in medical journals.

Biological changes associated with ageing are discussed in the language of abnormality and decay. Terms such as 'failing ovaries' and 'oestrogen deficiency' label the ageing women as diseased. So entrenched is the idea that the older woman is somehow diseased, that many women expect their minds and bodies to deteriorate after menopause.

In the British Columbia Office of Health Technology Assessment review of the evidence for selective BMD testing in Canada, the authors make this point:

> The effects of medicalisation on a social group can be far-reaching and subtle. For example, as natural phenomena become labelled as disease, anxiety is heightened. The general public is inundated about the 'discovered' disease. Social science research of medicine has repeatedly demonstrated how market forces may capitalise on a climate of risk and reassurance, which then drives the use of health technologies regardless of whether they lead to improved health outcome. This has been shown for ultrasound, electronic fetal monitors, predictive genetic screening, mammography, among others.[45]

There is a readiness to believe that if ageing is a disease, then it is a potentially curable one. The expected role of the physician is to assist in staving off this decline for as long as possible by offering regular screening to monitor the signs of decay, and treatment to avert diseases.

A recent article puts BMD testing in its social context:

> Once the fear of becoming diseased has been created, women are made to feel personally accountable for managing their risk of disease and future illness, and are encouraged to take appropriate measures to prevent it. Given that menopause has been defined in terms of hormone deficiency and osteoporosis increasingly defined in relation to that deficiency, any woman who wishes to avoid the 'diseases' of ageing will have to be tested for BMD and, if deficient, will have to embark on HRT.

. . . Individuals taking up this burden of preventing sickness and striving more and more to reach the ideal of normality may struggle in vain. The proliferation of disease categories and labels in medicine and psychiatry results in even more restricted definitions of 'normal'. This leads to increasing numbers of people being labelled abnormal, sick or deviant. The area of 'normality' is shrinking and the area of 'abnormality' or less than perfect health is increasing.[46]

Research of other cultures indicates that the menopause-associated decline is a uniquely western phenomenon. In many cultures the arrival of menopause signals a new freedom and increased social status where women gain increasing worth and veneration. Where the cultural expectation is to live a long and healthy life, it is self-fulfilling and individuals integrate that expectation and do live longer. In traditional Japanese society, for example, women expect to continue to be well; they become respected elders and fulfil a valued role in their communities. It has also been noted by anthropologists that menopause passes by unmarked biologically or socially in some cultures, particularly where frequent pregnancy and lactation is the norm, so that cessation of menstruation is relatively unremarkable.[47]

Osteoporosis and ageing

Many countries have not identified osteoporosis as a disease to be concerned about. Rates of fracture are very low in Africa, South America and most of Asia. In countries like Cambodia, it is reported to be unheard of.[48]

Gradual loss of bone density occurs naturally in all males and females with ageing, and at varying rates with different bones. Some bones actually gain density with age, and others lose very little mass. Age-related bone density loss does not as a matter of course equate with fragility fractures.

The weight of the establishment and the deeply entrenched idea that osteoporosis is reaching epidemic proportions make it difficult for anyone to seriously challenge the status quo. Women assume that their doctor is fully informed about the prevalence, diagnosis and treatment of osteoporosis, and don't realise that he or she is reliant upon the version of the story which has been imparted via drug company articles, glossy brochures, and industry-sponsored seminars and conferences which appear to have the full endorsement of the medical fraternity. Such is the powerful commercial infrastructure that has been built up around the osteoporosis industry that the illusion is complete. Virtually no one questions the appropriateness of widespread DXA screening, or the impact of a diagnosis of low bone density on a well woman. The unsuspecting patient and well-intentioned doctor are unaware in most cases that DXA screening is inaccurate, not a good predictor of fracture risk, and that front-line therapies for treating osteoporosis have serious associated risks and limited or non-existent evidence to support their effectiveness in preventing fracture.

Women are particularly easy to target because the medicalisation of menopause has paved the way for the medicalisation of bone mineral loss. A whole population of women in western countries has accepted they are at risk for a disease purely by virtue of their gender and reproductive status. Yet the evidence that every aspect of the disease is controversial and questionable and is largely commercially motivated is there for all to read in the medical literature — conveniently just out of reach of the popular pamphlets and posters produced by the big corporations that have a vested interest in perpetuating the fear and uncertainty.

The continuing power of the medical establishment is reflected in the naïve public perception that modern medicine and technology holds all the answers. But maybe it is time for a rethink. A recent article in the prestigious *Journal of the American Medical Association* confirmed that doctors are the third leading cause of death in the US, after cancer and heart disease. Every year 250,000 deaths result from medication errors, errors in hospitals, unnecessary surgery, and the negative effects of drugs. The author of the article, Barbara Starfield, on a recent visit to New Zealand, put the figures in context: prescription drugs alone claim 106,000 lives annually in the US. That is equivalent to three jumbo-jet crashes every two days.[49]

Bone and bone metabolism

Types of bone

Structurally, bone is of two types: trabecular bone and cortical bone.

Trabecular bone is the more porous honeycomb-like bone that forms the inner meshwork of the vertebrae, pelvis, flat bones and the ends of long bones. Trabecular bone constitutes only 20 percent of the skeleton but has a large surface area and is sensitive to metabolic changes. Trabecular tissue is the type of bone most subject to loss of density as we grow older, and to loss of structural integrity and strength with established osteoporosis.

Cortical or *compact bone*, which makes up 80 percent of the

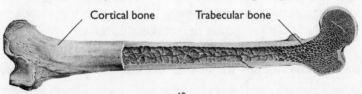

Cortical bone   Trabecular bone

skeleton, forms the outer casing of all bones and is the major constituent of the shaft of long bones.

The loss of bone that occurs with ageing can result in up to 35 percent reduction of cortical bone and as much as a 50 percent reduction of trabecular bone in women. Men lose approximately 25 percent and 35 percent of cortical and trabecular bone respectively.

Bone remodelling

Bone is made up of a framework or matrix of interlocking fibres of the protein collagen which forms the foundation for bone structure, and inorganic components which surround the collagen structure and form the 'cement'. Collagen is normally flexible and is important in the structure of skin and nails. In bone, however, it is made strong and rigid by tiny crystals of calcium phosphate salts being deposited on it. Calcium and phosphorus make the bones hard and strong, and collagen givens them their flexibility.

Bone is a living organ which is constantly remodelling, replacing and repairing itself. The adult skeleton is replaced entirely every 7–10 years. From birth to adolescence and to a lesser degree, young adulthood, there is massive bone remodelling going on as we grow taller and the long bones continue to extend. After the adolescent growth period ceases, the bone remodelling process slows, entering the maintenance phase, and then after menopause, most women appear to have higher levels of bone remodelling occurring again, although this can vary. In men, the age-related thinning of bones seems to occur about ten years later than it does in women.

The process of remodelling serves two purposes. Firstly, it keeps bones 'young'. Knock your leg, strain to pick up a heavy load, and the area of your bone which bears the impact will begin to repair the micro-damage which has occurred. The second purpose is to make bone better able to meet the regular demands placed upon it. This is why a violinist's bow arm, a TV person's camera-holding arm, or a racquet sport player's playing arm all develop bone that is thicker and stronger than the bone of the arm which has less expected of it.[1]

Bone is the only bodily organ that has cells designed specifically to destroy it. They are called *osteoclasts*. There are also cells called *osteoblasts* whose sole purpose it is to do the opposite, so healthy bones remodel and repair themselves in much the same way that road maintenance crews repair our damaged or weakened road surfaces. Bone is like a well-used highway which becomes cracked and worn with use and will eventually crumble unless the cracked and worn patches are removed and replaced. Bone remodelling occurs at sites where damage has occurred as a result of force as in a knock or fall, or when muscles have been working harder and applying greater pressure to bones. Breaking or cracking a bone generates an awe-inspiring sequence of events which will result in complete repair with new well-formed bone tissue. A certain amount of muscle strain is therefore a good thing in maintaining bone, and is the reason why exercise, particularly weight-bearing, is essential to perpetuate healthy bone remodelling.

The bone maintenance crews are called BMUs (basic multi-cellular units). About one million of these crews are working to remove and replace bone at any one time. When damage occurs in a patch of bone it is sensed by a network of cells called *osteocytes* which send signal molecules to alert the BMUs via an extensive 'osteo-internet'. As in road repair, the first members of the BMU to arrive are the diggers, the osteoclasts, which begin their process of removing bone. This process is known as resorption.

As the osteoclasts dig out the damaged patch, they actually release bone growth triggering factors which were left there 2–5 years earlier by the osteoblasts, whose purpose it is to rebuild the bone. These factors stimulate new osteoblasts to begin the rebuilding process. The osteoclasts have dug tunnels and trenches at the rate of about 0.0004 of a centimetre per day. Osteoblasts secrete collagen and laboriously fill in the excavated areas but take about eight times longer to do so. Gradually the new bone mineralises around the new web of collagen and after about 6–9 months the process is complete.

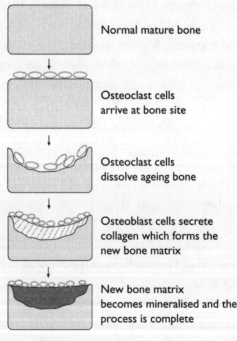

Normal mature bone

Osteoclast cells arrive at bone site

Osteoclast cells dissolve ageing bone

Osteoblast cells secrete collagen which forms the new bone matrix

New bone matrix becomes mineralised and the process is complete

The bone remodelling sequence.

At certain times of life, there is more bone building going on than remodelling — as in childhood and youth — so osteoblast cells predominate. Although the full story is not known, it seems that as we age, the BMUs are not as effective at patching and maintaining bone and we begin to lose more bone than we gain. It is believed that reduced bone density and osteoporosis occurs when many factors combine to produce BMUs with deeper-digging osteoclasts, and smaller crews of osteoblasts that cannot fill the bigger holes.

But the connection between bone formation and resorption is poorly understood at present, and is a key puzzle to be solved in the field of bone biology. When a person is identified with low bone density it doesn't automatically mean that they have reduced bone formation and greater bone resorption. Young people can have low bone density, and older people can have higher bone density.[2]

Dr Jane Aubin, specialist in anatomy and cell biology, and president of the prestigious American Society for Bone and Mineral Research, has spent much of her academic life studying what it is that causes osteoblasts to form. Interviewed in 1998 for an article in a Canadian women's magazine, she admitted that science's level of understanding of bone remodelling is at a basic stage. 'We are at the tip of the iceberg now . . . We don't even know what is in an osteoblast.'

The article also reports that the basic mechanisms of bone cell change are unknown. 'Dr Antonio Candeliere, one of Dr Aubin's postdoctoral fellows, added that he has no faith that a DXA measuring bone mass can tell you much of anything about the structural integrity of bone — whether or not a bone will fracture. "You've got to do a biopsy to study that."'[3]

Bone markers

In the bone remodelling process, certain chemical by-products are produced which can be found in blood and urine. Bone resorption produces certain types of chemicals, and the formation of bone produces others.

The chemicals produced during the bone remodelling process are called 'bone markers' and have become a relatively new addition to the osteoporosis diagnosis field. Bone markers can tell if a person's bone resorption is high or formation is low, and if treatment is embarked upon, can give some indication of its success after two or three months.

The accuracy of biochemical markers of bone turnover has improved markedly in the past few years, but there is still differing. opinion about their application. The general consensus is that measurement of bone turnover markers provides potentially useful information to supplement BMD measurement, but cannot be used to diagnose osteoporosis, evaluate its severity, or select a specific therapy.

There are markers that measure bone resorption and markers that measure bone formation.

Bone resorption markers

Dpd

The Dpd test measures levels of a substance called deoxypyridinoline or Dpd in urine. Dpd is the product of a type of collagen found in your bones which is excreted in urine as a result of the bone-breakdown process. It is a very specific marker of bone breakdown, and is unaffected by diet, making it suitable for assessing resorption. If you are not a young person and your Dpd measurement is high, then it could be an indicator that bone is being lost. At present it is not known whether it can be used to predict whether you are at risk for fracture.

Because bones remodel at a higher rate while you are sleeping, Dpd is measured from a urine sample collected from the first or second urination in the morning. A Dpd score of less than 6.5nM/mM is considered normal, based on the levels for healthy men and premenopausal women who are not pregnant. A score above 6.5 indicates rapid bone loss.

Collagen cross-links (NTX, CTX)

The activity of osteoclasts is measured by breakdown products of collagen. When bone is resorbed, collagen is broken down and fragments which contain the cross-linking molecules are released and excreted by the urine. High levels can indicate high levels of bone resorption.

Bone formation markers

Bone alkaline phosphatase (ALP)

Osteoblastic activity or bone formation is associated with osteocalcin, one of the proteins found in relatively high concentrations in bone. Bone alkaline phosphatase forms new calcium crystals, and blood levels of this bone enzyme give an indication of new bone formation.

Propeptide of type I collagen (PICP)

Another relatively new test measures PICP which is also associated with the secretion of collagen. It has been shown to correlate with bone formation.

CHAPTER THREE

Fractures – the facts

FRACTURES RELATED TO BONE FRAGILITY TEND TO BE AT those sites that involve a higher percentage of the porous honeycomb-like trabecular bone found on the inside, rather than hard cortical material covering the outside of bone. This is the predominant bone type in the hip and spine particularly. Other sites that may have fragility fractures are the wrist and the ribs. Fractures of the skull, ankle and the long bones of the leg are not usually associated with osteoporosis.[1]

Wrist fractures

Fractures of the wrist (Colles' fractures) are included in the osteoporosis statistics as they are common in women from 50–70 years of age. The lifetime risk of a Colles' fracture has been estimated to be 15 percent in white women. Women in this age group begin to lose balance more often than younger women. Wrists break when women fall because they react swiftly enough to stretch out their arms. Older women don't have the same speed of reaction and are more likely to fall directly onto their hip. Fitness, agility and the speed of gait are also factors. Women who walk faster are more likely to have forward momentum, and if they fall they land on their wrists.

A Colles' fracture can occur with normal, high, or low bone density of the forearm.[2] It is possible that factors related more to bone geometry rather than bone density are linked to forearm fractures.[3]

Wrist fractures, although painful at the time, usually repair successfully and do not typically have a long-term effect on quality of life. Neither do they predict subsequent fractures of the hip or spine. They cannot therefore be described as debilitating or devastating, and hardly warrant long-term pharmaceutical therapy as a preventative measure. There is minimal evidence at this point that currently available medications will prevent wrist fracture.

Vertebral fractures

The frightening image of the woman with the dowager's hump has been used to good effect by those who have much to gain from the industry, but just how common is the condition? According to a very recent study of the evidence for fragility fractures in Australian women aged 50, the lifetime risk of a clinical spine fracture was 9.6 percent and the risk of more than one vertebral fracture was one third of that again.[4]

Fractures of the vertebrae involve many types, from mild to severe. Vertebrae don't usually break, so fracture is actually the wrong term in most cases. Vertebrae tend to compress or become deformed when bone tissue deteriorates with ageing.

The course of spinal osteoporosis is unpredictable, and a low bone density measurement does not predict future events. Most often vertebral deformities take the form of a loss of height as a result of compression, without any associated pain or major symptoms. Loss of height may occur suddenly, or gradually over time. Most people are unaware that compression has occurred and 'fractures' are only revealed when found incidentally on X-ray. Wedging of vertebrae causing curvature in the spine can occur normally to some degree with ageing and is not necessarily associated with marked bone loss or fragility.[5] Loss of height may also be due to thinning of the cartilage discs between the vertebrae.

DXA scanning in its current form is not precise enough to identify spinal deformity; this can only be determined by radiographic assessment (X-ray) followed by careful measurement. Even then, the degree of compression of the vertebra necessary to define an actual clinical vertebral fracture is not standardised so statistics can vary widely. A height loss of more than 4 cm over 10 years has been used as a clinical marker of vertebral fracture.[6]

For research purposes, vertebral fractures are determined by measuring the height and width of the individual vertebra and comparing them to reference ranges. If the height has decreased by more than 3 standard deviations (or 20–25 percent) for that vertebra, it is deemed a fracture.[6]

In a minority of people, vertebral compression fractures may cause back pain which generally lasts a few months and can be managed with bed rest and analgesics. The fracture heals and normal life and activities can be resumed.[7] Spinal back pain may be due to compression fractures, but can also be due to other non-skeletal causes.[8]

In rare serious cases the vertebrae become wedge-shaped and an elderly woman may develop a hump in her back after multiple wedge 'fractures'. This is called *kyphosis* ('dowager's hump') and can bring chronic pain and other complications.

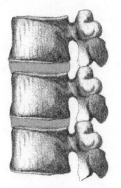

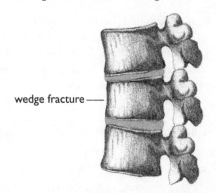

wedge fracture ——

Normal vertebrae.

Vertebrae that have begun to curve as a result of a mild wedge fracture.

Confusing statistics

Because there is no international standard for defining the degree of compression necessary to establish a vertebral fracture, there is wide variability in rates of fracture.

Dr Susan Ott comments: 'With vertebral fractures the incidence depends on how you measure the vertebra. If you define a fracture as only a small decrease in height then there will be a lot of them. If you use strict criteria, then there are not so many. Several studies have recently been reported showing how much difference it can make.'[9]

And even when the same criteria for defining a vertebral fracture is applied, the rates vary widely from one location to the next. In Europe, for example, the prevalence of deformities of the vertebrae shows enormous variation from country to country — as much as from six to 20 percent.[10] The highest rates are in Scandinavian countries.

Dr Bruce Ettinger, endocrinologist and osteoporosis expert, recently put the incidence of vertebral fracture in perspective:

> Clinical vertebral fractures are rare — vertebral deformities based on careful radiographic assessments are much more common. The incidence of the latter [deformities] is about 1 in 200 to 1 in 300 women per year. Clinical fractures are about $\frac{1}{3}$ of this rate. The 10 year risk of painful spine fracture for women at age 50 or at age 60 is very low, but the rate increases quite a bit with ageing.[11]

Despite these reasoned statements, hyperbole and frightening images continue to proliferate. A classic example of scaremongering is posted on the website of a well-known consultant gynaecologist from Chelsea & Westminster Hospital, London. This is the opening paragraph from his osteoporosis page:

> Osteoporotic fractures occur in one third of women, principally the hip (neck of femur), the vertebral bodies and the wrist. Apart from the life-threatening fracture of the hip which occurs in the older age group of women, the collapse fractures of the lumbar and thoracic vertebra produce pain, loss of height and the deformity of the dowager's hump. The capacity of the chest is diminished and women have their heart and lungs squashed up into small volume producing greater distress.[12]

Men and women have the same rate of fracture

Interestingly, the prevalence of spinal deformity appears to be much the same in men as it is in women under the age of 80 years. In a study of 16,119 European men and women aged 50–79, the incidence was 12 percent for males and 12 percent for females.[13] The same study showed an even higher incidence in younger men, which has led to speculation that some of the deformities were related to work-related accidents or trauma.

In a recent Canadian study men aged 50–59 years had a higher prevalence of spinal deformity than women the same age. But women tend to show more of an increase with age, and in the older age group — 80 years or more — 45 percent of women and 36 percent of men showed spinal *abnormalities* (not fractures).[14]

The spine consists of twenty-four vertebrae — each one cushioned by a flat cylindrical disk made from tough cartilage. The larger flat bone at the bottom of the vertebra is called the sacrum, and the tiny tail bone underneath the coccyx.

The spine is divided into three sections:

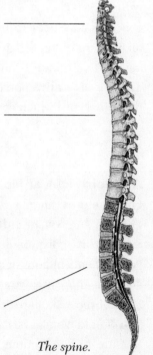

The cervical spine — the seven vertebrae at the top of the spine. They are generally less likely to be affected by osteoporosis.

The thoracic spine — twelve vertebrae in the middle of the back that have a pair of ribs attached to each of them. These bones are more prone to abnormality, and it is as a result of wedge fracture in the thoracic spine that the spinal 'hump' can be formed.

The lumbar spine — five vertebrae which are also susceptible to abnormalities.

The spine.

Treatment

Pain medication and rest will assist with the healing process after a vertebral compression fracture. When wedge and compression fractures have already occurred, pharmaceutical intervention in the form of the bisphosphonate Fosamax may help to prevent further fractures in a small percentage of patients, but the effectiveness and safety of long-term use is currently unknown. Hopefully treatments which meet acceptable criteria will be available in the near future.

Recently there has been interest in two 'minimally invasive' procedures for the management of acute vertebral fractures called *vertebroplasty* and *kyphoplasty*, which involve the injection of liquid plastic into the fractured vertebra. Reports with both techniques claim frequent acute pain relief. Some concerns have been expressed that the long-term effect of one or more reinforced rigid vertebrae on the risk of fracture of adjacent vertebrae is unknown for both of these procedures. There is also a five percent risk of 'leakage' of the plastic into the spinal cord which could cause serious damage.[15]

Hip fractures

A rational look at hip fracture statistics

Hip fractures, among all the fragility fractures, result in the greatest burden of suffering to the individual. While the evidence is indisputable that they are very serious and cost governments billions of dollars annually, it does not follow that all postmenopausal women are at risk for hip fracture.

Lifetime risk statistics are misleading and frightening. A 50-year-old woman has a 15 percent likelihood of having a hip fracture in her lifetime, and a man has a five to six percent risk.[16] This doesn't mean that once a woman is postmenopausal her risk is that high. The reality is that if you live until you are 90 years and if you are in poor health, your mind is not as sharp, your eyesight poor, your balance unstable and you are taking certain medications, there's a chance that you will fall down and break your hip. By the age of 90, about 17 percent of males have had a hip fracture, compared to 32 percent of females.

Much of the horror associated with hip fracture stems from the popular statistic that 20–30 percent of women who break a hip are dead within a year. The reality is that women who suffer a hip fracture and are relatively healthy rarely die from the fracture itself. It is estimated that as few as 14 percent of all deaths following a hip or pelvic fracture in women who were mobile before the event, were caused or hastened by the fracture. A recent UK study found that patients with depression, dementia or delirium appear to be at increased risk of death after hip fracture. Dr Holmes from the University of Leeds who conducted the study reported that the 'findings confirm what is not widely appreciated: that psychiatric illnesses have important effects on physical conditions'.[17]

A hip fracture is a very serious event and one that has a profound impact on quality of life, as evidenced by findings that 80 percent of women older than 75 years preferred death to a bad hip fracture resulting in nursing home placement.[18] But currently there is nothing a women in her 60s and 70s can do to avert fracture other than to stay fit and well, and avoid smoking and excessive alcohol intake. Hip fracture rates are comparatively high among elderly American, European and Australasian white women, low in most Asian women (other than Hong Kong Chinese and some urbanised Chinese), and low in African-Americans, African, Maori, Pacific Island and

Aboriginal women.[19, 20] A 1996 survey and assessment of hip fracture rates in Beijing found that they are among the lowest in the world but in situations of urbanisation may be rising rapidly.[21]

The vast majority of hip fractures occur after a fall, even though only one percent of all falls in the elderly result in a fracture. Only about 5 percent of hip fractures appear to be 'spontaneous' fractures, in which the patient fractures and then falls. The direction of the fall has a big part to play in the outcome. A fall to the side increases the risk of hip fracture by about six times, compared to falls in other directions. This is considered a much greater risk than lower bone density.[22]

Dr Susan Ott also comments: 'Other factors include how tall a patient is, how far she falls, how she lands, and maybe the shape of her hip. Also, factors that cannot be measured may be involved, such as how many of the bone cells are alive, how brittle the bone itself is, etc.'[23]

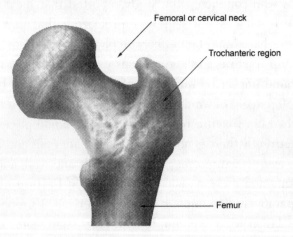

The hip or head of the femur. Fractures occur in the femoral neck or the trochanteric region.

Mechanical factors

At least half of all of hip fractures after the age of 80 are not directly linked to bone fragility, but rather are due to 'mechanical factors'. Common cervical fractures, or fractures of the femoral neck, appear to be more related to pelvic structure — failure of the outer diameter of the femoral neck to expand with age and 'increased acetabular bone width'. Women with trochanteric hip fractures (the wider area of bone at the head of the femur) have a more severe and generalised bone loss due to the greater amount of trabecular bone in that region of the hip.[24] Overall, about half of hip fractures are intertrochanteric and the others are femoral neck fractures. In older women the proportion of trochanteric fractures increases.

It is now recognised that hip fracture is a function not just of bone density but of the way people fall, of patterns of how weight on the hip is loaded (for example squatting), and of such structural features as hip axis length.[25] Many of these aspects vary across cultures. For example, hip fracture risk doubles with each standard deviation increase in hip axis length. Asian adults have shorter hip axes than adult Caucasians and, for the same bone mass, a lower hip fracture risk.

Treatments

There is no evidence that any of the available osteoporosis drug therapies will prevent hip fracture in the very elderly. As drugs are unlikely to address the major risk factors for hip fracture anyway, it makes much more sense to consider lifestyle and environmental factors.

These are:

- Maintaining body weight
- Walking for exercise, remaining active

- Exercises to increase balance and flexibility
- Avoiding long-acting benzodiazepines, corticosteroids, sleeping pills, etc.
- Minimising caffeine intake
- Treating impaired vision
- Removing potential tripping objects in the home
- Nourishment from a balanced nutrient-rich diet
- Exposure to sunlight.

Hip pads

In particularly frail elderly people who are at high risk for fracture, the wearing of a padded undergarment could help. A recent study found that the frail at-risk group who wore the underwear which incorporated a soft thin pad over each hip bone experienced five times more falls than the healthier less-at-risk control group, but had no fractures at all. The control group had a 4.3 percent fracture rate.[26]

The hip pads work on a principle similar to that of an automotive air bag. By first absorbing the shock of a fall, then dispersing its impact over a larger area, the padding reduces the damaging impact force of a fall on the vulnerable hip. Not surprisingly, they are not popular with many elderly people, so compliance with what could be an effective strategy is limited.

Summary

The evidence is conclusive that the greatest suffering comes about as the result of hip fractures in the elderly. Attention needs to be directed more to preventing such falls and to ensuring adequate nutrition and, where possible, minimal medication.

Without wishing to diminish in any way the seriousness of multiple wedge fractures of the spine, or the potentially devastating impact of hip fractures in old age, it is important to recognise that fracture statistics when presented in terms of lifetime risk are often misleading and needlessly alarming. Bone density loss occurs naturally with age, but as we have seen, not everybody develops thin and brittle bones. Neither are all postmenopausal women at risk for hip fracture. When the statistics for hip fractures are presented in the negative they present a dramatically different picture: 85 percent of women aged 50 with a life expectancy of 80 years will *not* suffer a hip fracture.

CHAPTER FOUR

Doubtful diagnoses

OSTEOPOROSIS IS A COMPLEX CONDITION WHICH IS STILL not fully understood. Diagnosis is therefore not as simple as it may appear. A diagnosis of osteoporosis can only really be established once there has been a fracture as the result of low impact or low trauma, which is confirmation that bone fragility exists. In the absence of fractures, osteoporosis is invisible and painless. There is as yet no way to accurately predict whether a person who has not yet fractured will fracture.

Because bone density measurement is a modern phenomenon, we have no idea what the bone densities of our parents or grandparents were like as they grew up, or even what our own were like as children. It is therefore difficult to define what is normal over a person's lifetime. Because of the short duration of good studies in the area, and only recent availability of relatively accurate methods for testing bone mineral density, there are still big gaps in the understanding of what is the natural history of bone formation and maintenance over a lifespan. With the availability of bone scanning technology, we are able now to measure the bone density of young people. But this raises many questions about current understandings of what is normal. For example, based on the World Health Organisation (WHO) definition of osteoporosis, only 84 percent of young people in America are reaching normal levels of bone density.[1]

The 1994 WHO definition which characterises osteoporosis as a measure of bone mineral density (BMD) has been largely adopted throughout the world because BMD is the easiest of the osteoporosis risk factors to measure. Bone mineral density has thus become the default definition of osteoporosis, which effectively means that one of the many risk factors has become the disease. As a consequence, all the research, treatment and preventative approaches are focused on BMD, and screening and diagnosing of healthy women continues to increase, despite widespread discrediting of its ability to predict fracture risk.

The initiation of BMD testing represents the entry point into the medical management of BMD. Now doctors can assume responsibility for monitoring and managing the density of their patients' bones from the first DXA scan until the end of their life. The availability of DXA technology has allowed physicians to begin to identify variations in bone mineral density amongst populations, and to observe changes in an individual over time, but these observations are of limited value if they don't help to prevent fragility fractures and reduce the incidence of osteoporosis. Doctors have the dilemma of determining whether low bone density puts their patient at risk or not, and whether they should be treated.

A recent Canadian Technology Assessment Review of the effectiveness of BMD testing warns:

A program which exposes a large segment of the population to lifelong medical attempts to maximise BMD should be required to justify these strategies on the basis of research evidence demonstrating that medical management can alter the natural history of fragility fractures.[2]

The same review of the evidence concluded:

Even the most favourable reports on the effectiveness of bone mineral testing reveal that BMD testing does *not* accurately identify women who will go on to fracture as they age.[3]

Bone density is only part of the story

The WHO describes osteoporosis as 'a progressive systemic skeletal disease, characterised by low bone mass and micro-architectural deterioration of bone tissue, with a consequent increase in bone fragility and susceptibility to fracture'.[4]

This definition identifies two main risk factors — loss of bone quantity, and loss of bone quality. DXA scanning measures only bone quantity (bone density or mass), not bone strength. Bone strength is determined by its micro-architecture, its size, shape, trabecular cross-bracing, and ability to repair damage. But because of perceived difficulties in measuring micro-architecture that whole aspect of bone health seems to be ignored, and bone density alone has become the focus of research and the definition of osteoporosis.

R. P. Heaney, international expert in osteoporosis, states:

The current prominence of BMD is due to the fact that it can be accurately measured and to some extent controlled. Indeed, essentially all preventative and therapeutic approaches to osteoporosis focus explicitly on acquiring and maintaining bone mass or on restoring lost mass. However, low bone mass probably accounts for less than half of all osteoporotic fractures. Thus history of fracture after age 40 and maternal history of hip fracture are stronger predictors than BMD and are independent of BMD.[5]

What the books, brochures and magazines don't tend to tell us is that a BMD measurement doesn't reveal information about bone micro-architecture. Nobody can tell from looking at a DXA scan or an X-ray, what a person's bone quality or strength is like. An invasive bone biopsy can give more of an idea, but for obvious reasons, this is not a popular procedure. At this stage we do not have the technology to be able to estimate bone strength. Therefore, a person can be low in bone mass but have perfectly normal bone structure.

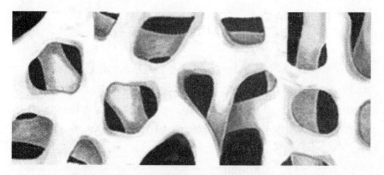

Microscopic image of normal trabecular bone.

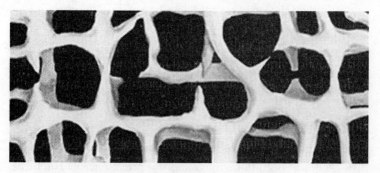

Image of weakened fragile osteoporotic bone.
This is not identifiable from a DXA scan.

With severe osteoporosis, the meshed, interlinked trabecular bone can erode, greatly weakening the bone. But a DXA scan is not able to identify this type of damage. Typically, literature on osteoporosis includes pictures for the edification of the patient depicting the various stages of osteoporosis. They show, as the disease progresses, the increasingly fragile and space-filled lacy network of disconnected trabecular bone, which looks as though it would disintegrate with the slightest of knocks. As patients are given a diagnosis of osteopenia, or osteoporosis, when these same labels are applied to the pictures of bone then it implies that these are images from a DXA scan.

The newly diagnosed patient is given every reason to believe that the pictures of osteoporotic bone accurately illustrate their diagnosis. In reality these popular images are taken from biopsies or autopsies, in most cases from people of advanced years.

Dr Susan Ott comments:

> Bone quality is determined by bone mass (as measured by bone density) and also by the micro-architecture of bone, the crystal size and shape, the brittleness, the connectivity of the trabecular network, the vitality of the bone cells, ability to repair micro-cracks, and the structure of the bone proteins. The fat cells, vasculature, neuronal pathways and bone marrow cells probably also influence the quality of the bone as well as the quantity of bone.[6]

The range of normal bone mineral density

In addition, there are significant and unexplained racial differences in both bone mass and the prevalence of fractures. If low bone mass is linked to fracture then we would expect to see more fractures in ethnic groups that have naturally low bone density. This is not the case. While it is true that people of African descent have higher bone mass and lower rates of fractures, it also happens that Asian women have lower bone mass than Caucasian women, but the rate of hip fractures is not proportionally higher. Hispanic women have approximately half as many fractures as Caucasian women, but their bone density is no different.[7]

In Malmo in Sweden there is a very high recorded rate of hip fracture — much higher than other western countries. But a study of the bone mineral density of this population found little evidence that low BMD was the cause. The authors of a study of this phenomenon reported:

> The Malmo bone mineral content was on the same level as in the United States, but higher than in Japan and France. The comparatively high level of fragility fractures in the Scandinavian countries cannot be explained by low bone mass.[8]

Falling is the big problem with the elderly, not bone density. Because any bone will fracture under certain conditions, a review of 28 studies concluded that most elderly women would fracture with the impact of an unprotected fall. The authors conclude:

> Differences in bone density between individual women are not great enough to discriminate between who will and who will not later suffer a fracture; this will be determined by chance, by conditions that increase the risk of falling or cause loss of the normal protective reflexes, and by illness and immobility causing bone loss shortly before the fracture.[9]

A similar consideration of the role of BMD testing in identifying vertebral fractures led to this conclusion:

> Our knowledge of the incidence and natural course of vertebral fractures and the effectiveness of preventive measures is limited, and with this uncertainty screening for vertebral body fractures cannot at present be recommended.[10]

Measuring a man's BMD using DXA scanning is also problematic. Applying the same standard of peak bone mass to the male skeleton as the female is probably inappropriate. Men generally have taller and larger skeletons than women and because DXA adjusts for the area scanned but doesn't completely correct for the fact that wider bones are also thicker, bigger bones appear to have greater BMD even if the actual tissue density of bone is no different.[11]

And the more elderly the person, the more difficult it is to accurately measure bone density. Dr Alan Tenenhouse, the principal investigator with the Canadian Multicentre Osteoporosis Study (CaMos) says that 'measuring bone mineral density of lumbar spine in the elderly, particularly men, is next to useless'.[12] This is because compression fractures, arthritis and the like, can cause artificially dense bone in the vertebrae of elderly people.

Bone densitometry testing

In 1988 Dual X-ray Absorptiometry (DXA) machinery was developed and quickly became the accepted gold standard technology to measure bone mineral density (BMD) because of its speed, safety and perceived accuracy. DXA is sophisticated computerised technology which, in a matter of minutes, and with minimal radiation exposure, can measure the mineral content of the vertebrae, the hip, the forearm, or even the whole skeleton. It prints out an impressive computer graphic of the bones it has scanned and tells you where your bone mineral density falls in relation to the set population 'normal'. DXA measures the bone mineral content (BMC) then divides that by the surface area of the bone that is being measured to create a BMD measurement in terms of grams per square centimetre. This has limitations as it provides only a two-dimensional reading, not three-dimensional measurement as many doctors believe it does.

The WHO definition cites BMD or BMC results as being equally or independently reliable in predicting osteoporosis (low bone density). But the prevalence of osteoporosis depends entirely upon the way in which DXA results are interpreted and expressed. For example, the prevalence of osteoporosis in the spine in women aged 70 years has been found to be approximately 30 percent when measured in terms of BMD, but is only half of that when BMC is used.[13]

Dr S. Pors Neilson discusses this in his recent article 'The fallacy of BMD: a critical review of the diagnostic use of dual X-ray absorptiometry':

> This fact is well known but is largely neglected. This neglect has the obvious consequence that osteoporosis is overdiagnosed in persons of petite body stature, simply because the means of reference populations are calculated from the values of large and small people.[14]

Accuracy and precision

The technical accuracy and precision of BMD measurements are considered by some to be barely satisfactory for clinical use. An accurate measurement would represent the true value of the mineral content of the targeted bone site. But error for DXA can be up to 8 percent in routine use. This means that the true value of a woman's bone density could be 8 percent higher or lower than what is reported to her. That is equal to almost one standard deviation.[15]

Precision refers to whether or not the same bone site can be measured repeatedly with an identical outcome. In the absence of international standards, DXA machines are calibrated differently, so precision is far from guaranteed. For this reason it is important to always be measured using the same machine which is using the same reference ranges, in follow-up testing.

Quantitative ultrasound

QUS or ultrasound offers a cheaper, more accessible method of bone density testing and is sometimes available in pharmacies and in doctors' surgeries. It uses sound waves rather than X-rays, and tends to most commonly measure the calcaneous or heel bone as it is limited to bone with minimal overlying soft tissue. It is a cheaper method of testing and is considered a reasonably useful diagnostic tool, but the results cannot be directly compared with the results of a DXA scan which remains the industry standard. It is not fully understood exactly what is being measured with heel ultrasound but it appears to be bone density and also properties of collagen in the bone, which is an aspect of micro-architecture. In this regard, it offers different information from DXA, but similarly doesn't accurately predict fragility fracture.[16]

Establishing normal peak bone mass

DXA measures the bone mineral density of an individual and then 'grades' it against an average peak bone mass which has been established from a selected young reference population. But as researchers are finding, peak bone mass varies widely from region to region, by gender, and even fluctuates seasonally. A Mexican survey of more than 4,000 healthy young people showed wide regional variations in peak bone density, and a recent Canadian study revealed the same inconsistencies.[17] As a consequence, concerned scientists and osteoporosis experts are warning that the technology may be diagnosing 'low bone density' when it is a normal level for that person, and a level which may never result in a fracture.

What is peak bone mass?

Adolescence is a crucial time for bone development. Surges in growth and in reproductive hormones initiate a spurt in bone growth which is responsible for almost half the adult bone mass. Peak bone mass (PBM) usually occurs somewhere around age 20 and is the total bone mass that a young person has after they have completed the growth of their long bones. The level of peak bone mass achieved in any individual is a reflection of all the things that have happened to the skeleton from its formation in the uterus through the years of growth into young adult existence. It is the sum of genetic and environmental factors. Once peak bone mass is achieved, bone mass tends to remain stable in both males and females until their late thirties and forties. After this time it begins to decline, at different rates for different individuals, and in different sites in the body. Bone density is, on average, lower in women than in men, but there is a wide range among individuals. Women on average lose between a third and a half of their peak bone mass over their lifetime while men lose less.[18]

It is believed that genetic factors account for an estimated 60–80 percent of the variability in PBM, with diet, physical activity and hormonal status being important factors as well.[19]

Some bones continue to grow. The skull increases in mass throughout life, and certain bones, the femur (thigh bone) and vertebrae for example, continue to increase in diameter as we get older. But it is generally agreed that the greater the peak bone mass achieved in youth, the greater protection a person has against fracture later in life when bone density progressively decreases for everyone.

At the time of writing, the natural history of bone development before menopause is particularly poorly understood because of a lack of longitudinal studies (studies over time) with good methodology and design. If the development of bone mass was better understood, then it is possible that strategies to build adequate bone in young people could be developed and tested. Once peak bone mass has been reached there are currently very limited options, if any, for reclaiming lost bone once fracturing occurs.[20]

In general, bone physiology is considered similar in males and females. A recent study showed that males have larger bones, but not necessarily stronger ones. The trabecular bone density is the same in males and females, and decreases with age in both. Whether DXA scanning using the same criteria for diagnosis is as relevant for men as it is for women is under debate. Generally, the criteria established for women is applied in the same way to men.

Manufacturers' reference standards

When you have your bone density measured by a DXA machine, you are given a computerised analysis which tells you whether your bone density is normal, or above or below normal. 'Normal' is a level that is set in the software of the DXA machine. If you are more than one standard deviation (SD) below that, then you are classified as abnormal.

What most people don't realise is that it is not their personal normal peak bone mass or their own age group's that they are being measured against, but that of a selected group of young 'normal individuals', which has been established by the DXA manufacturer in the United States. The WHO definition of osteoporosis recommends all women be measured and diagnosed using a young reference normal (T-score). A Z-score is when you are measured against an average BMD for your age and gender, but this is not used formally to diagnose.

Here is the surprising thing: *there is no agreed international reference standard, and each manufacturer has established their own independent average young normal data, resulting in vastly different standards between brands of DXA machines!*

There are three US manufacturers of DXA machines: Hologic, Lunar, and Norland. Their young normal reference standards have been created by measuring the peak bone mass of healthy young white women aged 20–29, or 20–39, or even up to the age of 50 years. Lunar reports that their reference data was obtained from 3,000 US and Northern European females, 1,400 French females, and 1,400 Japanese females.[21]

Although their original studies have not been made available for scrutiny, it is known that Hologic drew its reference subjects from the University of California in San Diego. It is believed that they were not a random sample of population but were chosen because they were exceptionally healthy, so they do not represent a normal young healthy adult. Screening in this way can create an artificially high 'normal' or mean peak bone mass which inevitably leads to biased results. Under these conditions many more people will be found to have low bone density and will consequently be given a diagnosis of osteoporosis.[22]

During the course of their review, the authors of the British Columbia Office of Health Technology Assessment study contacted the manufacturers of DXA machines directly to find out how the subjects were selected, but other than gross indications for exclusion such as medication, substance abuse and illness, were given very little information about important factors like age, nutrition, exercise patterns, or even weight and height of the individuals used. They add: 'We have no assurance that the range of "young normals" were not biased by the inclusion of a disproportionately large number of athletic team members.'[23]

Evidence that manufacturers' standards are unreliable

More recently, concerned researchers in various countries have established their own young normal standards based on local populations and have invariably found them to be different from the US manufacturers' — usually much lower. When they have applied their own local young normal reference standards for general screening instead of the manufacturer's, the outcomes have been very different as well — suggesting that massive variations in diagnosis are taking place, dependent entirely upon which country or which machine is doing the measuring.

Two large studies, one in the US and one in Canada, measured local population samples of young people in order to set their own DXA reference standards. They then measured a large cross-section of the population using their local standard, and compared this with the manufacturer's standard.

The first study, the third National Health and Nutrition Examination Survey (NHANES III) chose a sample of young women who were more diverse in terms of body size and other environmental factors than the manufacturer's group. The authors say they did this deliberately because they wanted the reference group to reflect a normal BMD level — one that actually exists in the population.[24] The result was an average peak bone mass which was much lower than that set by the DXA companies; this cut the prevalence of osteoporosis as defined by BMD by more than half. For example, if they had used the manufacturer's reference range in their study, the prevalence of osteoporosis in the hip would have been 49 percent rather than the 28 percent that they identified.[25]

The second, a very recent Canadian government-funded epidemiological study of 10,000 people (see graph on page 76), set its own population-specific reference standard using a random selection of young women and came up with equally astonishing results. They found the actual prevalence of osteoporosis (as defined by low bone density) to be 16 percent in women and 5 percent in men, as opposed to the official Canadian estimates of 50 percent and 12 percent. Established fracture rates in the study population were also comparatively low. Only 10 percent of women in their study who were over 50 years had fractured, and most of those fractures were of the small bones and feet. There were only occasional serious fractures in areas such as the hip or the pelvis.[26, 27]

There were similarities between the US and Canadian outcomes. When the researchers of the Canadian study applied the NHANES III criteria for the hip and compared it to the Canadian criteria, the outcomes were almost the same. When they were compared with the manufacturer's criteria, however, the outcome was vastly different.

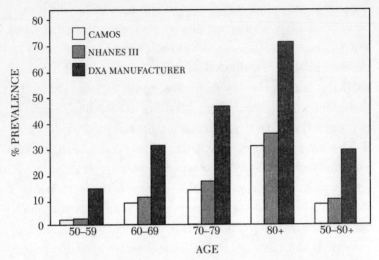

Incidence of osteoporosis (low bone density) in the hip in
Canadian women. A comparison of Canadian (CAMOS), US
(NHANES III) and DXA manufacturer's reference standards.
Source: A Tenenhouse. *Osteoporosis International 2000.*
Reproduced with permission.

Another very recent study from Turkey shows the prevalence of
low BMD fell from 50.3 percent to 14.0 percent at the spine,
and from 60.8 percent to 14.6 percent at the hip, when the US
manufacturer's standard was compared with a locally produced
standard.[28] The authors conclude by saying, '. . . our data suggests that individual populations should use their own reference
range T-scores in DXA in order to avoid misdiagnoses of
osteopenia and osteoporosis based on other populations'
reference range T-scores. Since a low normal BMD is not
necessarily indicative of an increased risk of fracture in a given
population, this approach might decrease unnecessary patient
anxiety and errors concerning treatment.'

In a study from the UK published in 1997, the bone mineral densities of 2068 women aged 30–70 were measured. Fifty-four percent were in the normal range according to a locally determined standard but only 25 percent were normal against the manufacturer's standard, leading the researchers to comment: 'We observe that manufacturers' reference ranges may not be appropriate for the local population and may lead to an erroneously high diagnosis of osteopenia and osteoporosis, which would lead to unnecessary patient anxiety and perhaps errors regarding treatment'.[29]

Another UK study reports: 'Our findings suggest that patients may be diagnosed as having osteoporosis if one reference range is used but not if another is used, even when the same manufacturer's dual-energy X-ray absorptiometry system is used.'[30]

Not surprisingly, some experts are beginning to question the relevance and accuracy of current standards for DXA scanning and the WHO criteria.[31, 32, 33] Even correcting the situation is not simple. They also warn that any updates or changes planned to overcome this major problem could make it very difficult to interpret previous readings.[34]

In the main, doctors and general practitioners who recommend bone scanning to their patients are unaware of or are confused by the controversy, and trustingly make decisions on the basis of the outcome of the DXA scan.

The massive discrepancies in the diagnosis of osteoporosis resulting from inconsistent and inaccurate DXA scanning raise serious concerns that many people are being diagnosed with osteoporosis and then treated with prescription medications when they will never have a fragility fracture.

New Zealand's story

The use of DXA screening has increased exponentially in the last decade. In New Zealand there were two such devices in 1992, used mainly for research purposes; now there are at least thirty spread over the country's main centres. Machines such as these cost an average of US$150,000 each and a screening appointment in NZ costs a patient between $65 and $150 each visit.

A phone survey of the laboratories offering BMD screening in NZ revealed all three brands of machines (Hologic, Lunar and Norland) are in use, and although some of the technician-operators were uncertain of specifications, most appear to be calibrated to the manufacturer's standards. Norland offer a US standard for the measurement of Maori and Pacific Island women, an Australian standard for Pakeha (white) New Zealanders, and a Japanese standard for Asian clients. Most, but not all, of the Hologic machines have had their software upgraded to now include the internationally recommended NHANES III reference data for the hip. At this time there is no such standard for the spine.

There is no standardisation between manufacturers, and reference data can vary widely from one centre to another. As one osteoporosis expert puts it: 'Different machines give different results even at the same site and with similar technology. For example, values for BMD at the lumbar [lower] spine using Hologic DXA give values . . . lower than values using the Lunar machine. This difference (approximately 10 percent) is roughly equivalent to a standard deviation of the population range of BMD.'[35] This means that it is possible for a NZ woman (or any woman, anywhere) to have her bones scanned in one laboratory and have a diagnosis of low bone density, then go elsewhere to have the same procedure on a different brand of machine and be told that she is normal.

An Australian representative of one of the manufacturers was contacted to discuss this point and she confirmed that diagnosis was inconsistent and widely varying from laboratory to laboratory. She was quick to reassure, however, that over-diagnosis, should it occur, could only be a good thing, remarking: 'Wouldn't you rather be told you have osteoporosis even if you don't so that you can take preventative action?'[36]

A 1990 NZ study of 462 women and 264 men from one geographical location, ranging in ages from 20–84, found that NZ postmenopausal women had *higher* bone density at the spine (but not the hip) when compared with other normal populations.[37] This study, which used now obsolete technology, has been cited as a justification for not replacing the DXA manufacturers' standards with local reference standards, and for accepting the higher manufacturer's standard as 'good enough'.

Rather mystifyingly, we are advised that osteoporosis is a major health issue in NZ, with 56 percent of all postmenopausal women predicted to have an osteoporosis-related fracture. If bone density is reported to be naturally higher in this population, and high bone density is claimed to be protective against fracture, it is curious that fracture estimates are also very high for postmenopausal women in this country.

The toll on the patient

The psychological effects of being labelled abnormal or at risk are rarely considered. Such labels cause great distress and anxiety and are known to 'affect the identity and shape the life experience of those who are so labelled'.[38] My years as a meno-pause educator have confirmed the prevailing fear that many women have of developing osteoporosis. Their doctors routinely recommend BMD testing as part of the menopause 'wellness' package, and once such testing is embarked upon, they are invariably caught in the re-screening loop. An abnormal diagnosis requires repeat testing which leads to increasing dependency on BMD testing. HRT and other pharmaceuticals are also likely to be administered over many years in order to ensure that women retain 'normal' levels of bone density.

> Susie looked very anxious as she told her story. She had had an early menopause, had used HRT for a few months only, then managed the rather difficult transition with exercise and herbal treatments. Now ten years on at age 48 she had been recommended a bone density test because she was told her early menopause put her at greater risk for osteoporosis. Her bone density measured as normal, but she was still very worried. Although it was normal, it was at the low end of normal. Because she believed that she was on the brink of rapid age-related bone loss, she thought the result meant she was still at serious risk for fracture. Neither could she be reassured. She was convinced by information from her doctor and the computerised print-out from the DXA machine that her bone mass was about to slip from the 'normal' range into the 'diseased' category.

Accuracy of diagnosis is imperative as younger women of menopausal years who are identified as having low bone mass in the spine are likely to be encouraged to embark upon treatment which to be useful must be taken long term. Women are told that for HRT to provide protection against further bone loss and fracture, long-term compliance is essential, typically over several decades.[39] This is something that most women would rather not do, as it exposes them to the ongoing increased risk of breast cancer and other serious complications.

Postmenopausal women report that the results of bone densitometry substantially influence their decision to begin hormone replacement therapy. A study found that women with moderate low bone loss were twice as likely to start HRT as women with normal bone mass, and women with severe low bone mass are more than three times as likely to start.[40]

BMD testing — further limitations

Bone mineral density testing has other limitations too. The sites most commonly measured are the hip and the spine. But your bone density can vary throughout the skeleton, so it is hardly conclusive that you have osteoporosis when one part of you, say the lower spine, registers as having low bone density, because the hip may be normal, or vice versa. The NHANES III study found that even different parts of the hip resulted in vastly different measurements. For example, only 10 percent of the population studied had osteoporosis in the whole hip (femur) region, whereas 17–20 percent had osteoporosis when each region of the hip was considered separately. In one group of women 17 percent would have been classified as having osteoporosis in terms of the WHO criteria after having just the neck of the femur scanned, but only six percent would have osteoporosis when the entire hip region was scanned.[41]

In the same study, the bone densities of 351 women and 348 men ranging in age from 21 to 93 years were measured in 15 different body sites — including the spine, hip, wrist, leg, head, pelvis and ribs. Results differed considerably from one site to another, and from men to women. The areas with the lowest BMD were the lumbar spine, the hip and the wrist, although the stages in life when bone density was lost were quite different. Bone density in the hip, for example, began to decline very slowly from the age of 20, whereas spinal bone density was stable in women until menopause.[42]

What the independent analysts say

There are now over 20 agencies for health technology assessment worldwide, established by governments and organisations responsible for funding health care. These agencies provide rigorous and systematic reviews of the effectiveness of medical interventions to assist them to develop policies that will improve the health status of their country's populations. The reports are externally reviewed, and available to the public.

The Swedish Council on Technology Assessment in Health Care (SBU) was founded in 1987 while centres at York (NHS Centre for Reviews and Dissemination) and Canada (Canadian Coordinating Office for Health Technology Assessment) were established in the early 1990s.

Reports on bone mineral testing and associated treatments have been furnished by 14 of these agencies. The British Columbia Office of Health Technology Assessment analysis of the findings of fourteen major systematic review groups concluded that BMD testing does not result in a reduction of fractures, and is therefore not a cost-effective public health strategy.

The following are statements on the usefulness of bone density testing from some of those agencies:

The British Columbia Office of Health Technology Assessment:[43]

Clinical management decisions should not be altered by BMD test results, except in instances where BMD test results may help in the diagnosis of women with symptomatic conditions. In particular, BMD testing should not be used to assist in decisions regarding preventive strategies such as hormone therapy [HRT], nor should it be used to establish a risk assessment of well women. In both of the latter instances, BMD test result will mislabel women more often than not.

The Alberta Heritage Foundation for Medical Research:[44]

There will be substantial numbers of false positives [i.e. diagnoses of osteoporosis] and false negatives [normal when not] when bone density measurement (BDM) is used to assess whether or not an individual is osteoporotic on the basis of the WHO definitions. Many women will be assigned to the wrong category for their risk of fracture.

University of Newcastle Osteoporosis Study Group, Australia:[45]

The measurement of BMD is not a useful screening test for the identification of women at high risk of hip fracture and requiring preventative treatment with estrogens.

Agence Nationale pour le Développement de l'Evaluation Médicale, France:[46]

Bone mineral density measurement cannot be considered a good screening test (presence of false positives and false negatives decreasing the individual predictive value for fractures).

Swedish Council on Technology Assessment in Health Care:[47]

There is no scientific basis for recommending bone density measurement in mass screening, selective screening, or as an extra component in health check-ups of asymptomatic individuals (opportunistic screening).

And with reference to the evidence for national screening programmes:

The International Network of Agencies for Health Technology Assessment:[48]

> When all the scenarios are considered, a BMD screening program aimed at menopausal women might prevent between 1 percent and 7 percent of fractures. Taken together, these estimates of the effectiveness of such a program are not particularly encouraging from a public health perspective and are unlikely to represent good value for money.

Effective Health Care Bulletin, UK:[49]

> It is likely that a bone screening programme will lead to the prevention of no more than 5 percent of fractures in elderly women. Given the current evidence, it would be inadvisable to establish a routine population based bone screening programme for menopausal women with the aim of preventing fractures.

The substantial concerns raised by health technology assessment agencies on the effectiveness of bone density measurement and associated treatments warrant close consideration by those concerned with the management of osteoporosis, but to date they appear to have had little effect. The assessment had a temporary influence in public health policy in Canada, but the use of BMD screening advances remain unchecked in the rest of the western world.

A salutary tale

After the furnishing of the British Columbia Office of Health Technology Assessment report on the effectiveness of bone density screening in 1996, the Medical Services Commission there imposed a moratorium on public funding of bone densitometry (DXA) testing in new facilities in the province.

This effectively stopped the growth of BMD technology in publicly funded facilities in the province for three years. The Medical Consultant who chaired the BC Ministry of Health at the time was responsible for the moratorium, as he was convinced that there was no scientific evidence that BMD testing led to better patient outcome. But his actions were to cost him. As of late 1999, the contract of the Medical Consultant had not been renewed and he had subsequently left the ministry. The BMD moratorium ended and in 1999 the number of publicly funded facilities with BMD-testing capacity doubled. Commercial interests quickly took up their cause of promoting BMD testing in the province.[50]

Selective screening of well women

Some countries are encouraging doctors to select well women who seem to be more at risk for osteoporosis at the time of menopause and screen them, rather than all women at menopause. This is dependent of course upon the doctor being able to identify the woman who has a high risk of future fractures, *before* she fractures. As most fractures occur in women long after they have gone through menopause, and are due to factors which are not manifest at this time, there is no evidence to support selective screening either.[51]

The doctors' dilemma

Women accept the advice of their doctor in the belief that he or she is fully informed of the accuracy of methods of diagnosing osteoporosis, and the effectiveness and safety of treatment. Little do they realise that doctors are just as likely as they are to be influenced by the market forces which perpetuate the epidemic theory. Rather than doing their own literature searches, doctors are most often educated by drug company literature and seminars. As a consequence, many of them use bone mineral density testing widely, and go on to treat their patients on the basis of low BMD. Authors of the Alberta Technology Assessment Review comment that the significance and limitations of BMD results seem poorly understood in general practice.[52]

Concerns have also been raised about the interpretation of BMD results. A knowledge of statistics is required, and interpretations can vary from one laboratory and physician to another. A person with osteoporosis can be cared for by her GP, a gynaecologist, endocrinologist, or a rheumatologist, each with their own approach to assessing the condition.

The dilemma for physicians is to determine whether low bone density puts their patient at risk for fracture or not, and therefore whether to recommend treatment. Most doctors are not aware that evidence for a link between low BMD and fracture is minimal, and that they may do their patient greater harm by prescribing medication. It is hard to argue with the apparent objectivity of a machine — a glamorous one at that, offering a dazzling personalised printout. But consider this: the University of Leeds examination of the effectiveness of BMD screening found that of the 20 percent of women with the *lowest* bone density measurements only 28 *percent* of those would have gone on to fracture later. Women who registered with higher bone density would have 63 percent of all fractures![53]

CHAPTER FIVE

Risk factors for osteoporosis

ESTABLISHED OSTEOPOROSIS (WITH FRACTURE) CAN
have many causes. As a result there are many different
'types' of osteoporosis. Low bone density is just one of many
risk factors for fragile bones. A diagnosis of low bone density
can only accurately predict future fracture in a person who is
already deemed to be at high risk because of other factors.[1]

For example, a major factor often overlooked in people who
are considered 'normal', yet fracture easily, is the issue of
prescription drugs.[2] Physicians are sometimes unaware that
the drug they are prescribing can create bone fragility as a
side-effect and there is concern that doctors need to be more
aware of this problem when assessing their 'at risk' patients.
The list of drugs which can cause osteoporosis-related fracture is extensive, and given their widespread use could well
account for much of the incidence of fragility fractures in these
times.

Secondary causes

In any case where a person is identified as having low bone density as well as a history of fracturing, what are called secondary causes — other risk factors or conditions which bring about osteoporosis as a result — need to be investigated. In pre- and peri-menopausal (those undergoing menopause) women, more than 50 percent of osteoporosis is associated with secondary causes and the most common causes cited are low oestrogen levels (most often as the result of a removal of the ovaries), glucocorticoid drugs, thyroid hormone excess, and anticonvulsant therapy.[3]

In cases where young people fracture easily and have low bone mass, there is also very often a secondary cause. Many young people taking Prednisone and other glucocorticoids for asthma and other conditions are at risk. In a recent statement on osteoporosis from the US National Institutes of Health, concerns were raised about this issue and the need for development of glucocorticoids that avoid effects on the skeleton.[4]

In postmenopausal women, the prevalence of secondary conditions is thought to be lower, but in reality it is not known, as very often tests are not done to determine factors other than postmenopausal status. Diagnosis is commonly made on the basis of a BMD test alone. However, in one study of postmenopausal women, hypercalciuria (the excretion of abnormally large amounts of calcium in the urine), hyperparathyroidism (the overproduction of parathyroid hormone by the parathyroid glands) and malabsorption (poor absorption of nutrients via the digestive system) were identified. These women were found to have osteoporosis (low BMD) but otherwise had no history of conditions that cause bone loss.[5]

Osteoporosis in men is usually related more to secondary

causes such as excessive alcoholism, smoking, glucocorticoid treatments like Prednisone and cortisone for asthma, rheumatoid arthritis, inflammations, etc.[6] It is believed that 30 to 60 percent of osteoporosis in men is associated with secondary causes. In recent times attention has been given to low levels of the male hormones, testosterone in particular, which like oestrogen is implicated in bone loss. Testosterone increases muscle mass, which indirectly results in higher bone density. Testosterone is also converted to oestrogen, which in turn influences bone resorption.

In a recent study of 355 men over the age of 60, previous fractures, gastrectomy, peptic ulcer disease, rheumatoid arthritis, glucocorticoid use, hypertension, previous hyper-thyroidism, height loss since age 20 years, chronic lung disease and smoking were related to lower density.[7]

Other risk factors

Bone health in younger age groups — up to and around menopause — is determined by many factors. For example, a family history of fragility fracture, smoking, inadequate diet, a lack of exercise, certain medications and the presence of certain diseases may result in fragile bones.

Risk factors for older people are different and revolve around the increased propensity to fall. An elderly person is more likely to fall under the influence of certain medications, and multiple prescribing for a variety of complaints and the effect of drug interaction can compound the problem. Dementia, frailty and immobility along with low bone density further increase the risk.[8] In an often quoted study of 9,516 white women over the age of 65 which measured their risk factors for hip fracture, the following are listed as the most predictive factors:

- A maternal history of hip fracture
- Having the same body weight as at age 25
- Previous fractures after the age of 50
- Being tall at the age of 25
- Self-rated health being fair or poor
- Previous hyperthyroidism
- Medications — specifically sedatives, anti-depressants and long-acting benzodiazepines or anticonvulsant drugs
- Less than four hours a day on feet.[9]

Women with five or more of these risk factors, including low bone density in the heel, were more likely to have a hip fracture than women with no more than two, and normal bone density.[10] The authors conclude that maintaining body weight, walking for exercise, avoiding medications, minimising caffeine intake, and treating impaired visual function are among steps that may decrease risk.

An Australian study which set out to identify the risk factors for hip fracture among elderly men and women found that smoking, being underweight in old age, being overweight at age 20 and weight loss were linked to an increased risk for hip fracture. Consumption of dairy products, particularly at age 20, was associated with an *increased* risk of hip fracture in old age. Caffeine and alcohol intake were not associated.[11]

Medical conditions
A large number of medical conditions are associated with lowered bone density and increased risk of fracture. These fall into several categories:

- Hormone disorders such as hyperparathyroidism, hyper-thyroidism, hypothyroidism

- Gastrointestinal diseases such as celiac disease

- Blood disorders

- Genetic disorders

- Connective tissue disease such as rheumatoid arthritis

- Nutritional deficiencies

- A variety of other common serious chronic systemic disorders, such as congestive heart failure, end-stage renal disease, and alcoholism.

Because much of the osteoporosis research focuses on bone density alone, risk factors are frequently identified as those that are shown to increase bone density loss. When considering the following examples, therefore, it is good to remember that they are mostly discussing conditions or situations that influence bone density, which is itself one of many risk factors. In many cases research does not include fracture risk.

Thyroid conditions

Your thyroid is a small bowtie or butterfly-shaped gland located in your neck, wrapped around the windpipe below the Adam's apple area. The thyroid has the only cells in the body which are capable of absorbing iodine. It produces several hormones, of which two are key: triiodothyronine (T3) and thyroxine (T4). Once released by the thyroid, the T3 and T4 travel through the bloodstream. Their purpose is to help cells convert oxygen and stored calories into energy.

A woman faces as high as a one-in-five chance of developing thyroid problems during her lifetime. She may suffer from hyper- (too much) or hypo- (too little) thyroid hormones. That risk increases with age and for those with a family history of thyroid problems.

Hyperthyroidism

Hyperthyroidism is a well-known risk factor for osteoporosis caused by an excess of circulating thyroid hormone. Thyroid hormone activates osteoclasts and bone resorption. Hyperthyroidism is therefore associated with an increase in bone resorption and a decrease in bone mass. It is quite common, affecting about 2 percent of women and 0.2 percent of men. Treatment for hyperthyroidism can result in hypothyroidism.

Hypothyroidism

Most people with thyroid disease suffer from hypothyroidism. That is, they are not producing enough thyroid hormone. In this situation the thyroid is either underactive, totally unable to function, or has been surgically removed. There is evidence that women taking thyroid replacement (thyroxine) may also be at increased risk for excess bone loss, particularly if the dose of thyroxine is too high, or taken over many years. Careful regulation of thyroid replacement is important.[12]

Hyperparathyroidism

Though their names are similar, the thyroid and parathyroid glands are entirely separate glands, each producing distinct hormones with specific functions. The parathyroid glands are four pea-sized glands located on the thyroid gland in the neck.

The parathyroid glands secrete parathyroid hormone (PTH), a substance that helps maintain the correct balance of calcium and phosphorus in the body. PTH regulates release of the calcium from bone, absorption of calcium in the intestine, and excretion of calcium in the urine. When the amount of calcium in the blood falls too low, the parathyroid glands secrete just enough PTH to restore the balance.

If the glands secrete too much hormone, as in hyper-parathyroidism, the balance is disrupted and blood calcium rises. This condition of excessive calcium in the blood, called hypercalcemia, or in the urine (hypercalciuria) indicates that something may be wrong with the parathyroid glands. The excess PTH triggers the release of too much calcium into the bloodstream. As a result, the bones may lose calcium, and too much calcium may be absorbed from food. The levels of calcium may increase in the urine causing kidney stones. PTH also acts to lower blood phosphorus levels by increasing excretion of phosphorus in the urine.

Celiac disease

Celiac disease is a genetic disorder of the small bowel or the duodenum. In celiac disease, the digestive tract is damaged by gluten proteins from wheat and other grains and as a result does not effectively absorb nutrients including essential minerals for healthy bones. Celiac disease can account for a spectrum of illnesses ranging from relatively mild digestive symptoms to more serious conditions including established osteoporosis and intestinal cancer. It is often undiagnosed because of its range of mild and varied symptoms, but many of these including osteoporosis (low BMD) can be reversed effectively in most people when gluten is eliminated from the diet.

It is not known how many people have the disorder, but recent figures suggest that one in 300 people of European descent may be affected — many of these not being aware that they are. Simple blood tests that detect certain antibodies are effective ways of establishing whether you may have celiac disease. The antibody tests are endomysial, reticulin (IgA), and gliadin (IgG and IgA). Final confirmation is usually by way of a biopsy of the small bowel via gastroscopy, although full diagnosis through blood tests is close to being a reality.

It is possible that far more people have celiac disease and are intolerant of gluten than is known, because many physicians don't consider it in their elimination process. It is reasonable to conclude, therefore, that many seemingly healthy people may have correctable low bone density as a result of the disorder.

In a recent Italian study 86 newly diagnosed celiac disease patients, 66 percent of whom were found to have osteoporosis (low BMD) or osteopenia, adopted a gluten-free diet and then had their bones scanned again after one year. The diet led to significant improvement in bone mineral density, even in postmenopausal women.[13] Another study of Italian children and adolescents with newly diagnosed celiac disease and associated remarkably reduced bone density in the whole body, found that a one-year gluten-free diet lead to a complete remineralisation of their bones so that they had the same density as other young people without celiac disease.[14] Other studies in Scandanavia and Argentina have shown similar dramatic results.

Regular screening for celiac disease in people who are diagnosed with low BMD osteoporosis may therefore provide a relatively simple solution for many people. A gluten-free diet these days is not that difficult as alternative flours and palatable breads, pastas and baking are more readily available.

Vitamin D deficiency

Vitamin D (sometimes called a hormone and sometimes a

nutrient) helps to control the formation of bone tissue. It increases the amount of calcium and phosphorus the body absorbs from the small intestine and thus helps regulate the growth, hardening, and repair of the bones. It is essential for the normal growth and development of the teeth, bones, and cartilage in children. It is also needed to keep adult teeth in good repair.

There are two forms of vitamin D: ergocalciferol, which is found in a relatively small selection of foods such as herring, mackerel, salmon and halibut; and cholecalciferol, which the body manufactures when exposed to the sun. Vitamin D is fat-soluble, can build up inside the body, and therefore is highly toxic when taken in large doses for a long time.

Vitamin D prevents osteomalacia or rickets, a deficiency disease characterised by malformations of bones and teeth in children and by brittle, easily broken bones in adults. Age-related vitamin D deficiency leads to malabsorption of calcium, accelerated bone loss, and increased risk for hip fracture. Vitamin D supplementation with calcium has been found to retard bone loss and reduce hip fracture.[15] Low vitamin D levels can be determined from a blood test.

Sunlight exposure of the skin is known to be the most important source of vitamin D. Severe vitamin D deficiency is therefore prevalent amongst people who have insufficient exposure to the sun, including elderly people who may be institutionalised or confined indoors. A study of heavily veiled Moslem women living in Denmark found that they needed to supplement with at least three times the recommended daily amount in order to secure a normal level of 25-hydroxyvitamin D, the metabolite of vitamin D which circulates in the blood.[16]

With thinning of the ozone layer over countries in the

southern hemisphere like Australia and New Zealand there is a need to cover the skin to avoid sunburn and skin cancer, and it may be that vitamin D levels will be affected. The prevalence of vitamin D depletion in adults is believed to be on the increase.[17]

Lack of exercise

Regular weight-bearing exercise, once a natural part of life, has been abandoned by many for a more sedentary lifestyle. This translates directly into less dense bones. Astronauts lose bone density as soon as they become weightless. Well-controlled studies are showing that people who exercise three times a week can increase their bone density, compared to those who are sedentary and actually lose bone density.[18] And age is no barrier. People 80 years and over who exercise regularly reduce bone loss while also improving muscle tone and balance, which in turn reduces the risk of falling.[19] Exercise can also reduce the need for medications in some cases.

Menstrual irregularities in young women

Failure to achieve peak bone mass, bone loss, and increased fracture rates have been evident in young women who have abnormal patterns of menstruation. Low levels of female hormones in a young woman brought about by delayed start of menstruation, very few menstrual periods or an absence of menstrual periods, are relatively common in adolescent girls and young women. These can occur as a result of strenuous athletic training, emotional stress, and low body weight.

Weight loss

A cultural belief that thin-is-better has generated in some women a lifelong tendency to diet. Many well-controlled studies have shown that when a woman loses weight, regardless of age, she loses bone.[20] Women who exercise to the point of interrupting their menstrual cycle are known to lose bone density and even to fracture.[21]

Eating disorders

Anorexia nervosa and bulimia are conditions which particularly affect young people, and can have devastating consequences. They usually involve an abnormal fear of obesity, a distorted body image, and abnormal eating patterns such as obsessive fasting, self-induced vomiting or the use of laxatives. The effects of these disorders range from mild weight loss to delayed sexual development, heart problems, depression, osteoporosis (low bone density) and even death.

Research has indicated that the condition might result in bone mass loss in up to 90 percent of anorexic women. Tests of 130 young women with anorexia showed that 38 percent of them had osteoporosis as defined by bone mineral density. The researchers from the General Hospital in Massachusetts indicated that 92 percent of the women showed bone mass loss at the hip, the spine and the extremities. The research indicated that supplementary female hormones (HRT) did not reduce the risk of bone mass loss in these women.[22]

The investigators conclude that in these women body weight, not oestrogen deficiency, is a significant predictor of bone mineral density, and stress that anorexic women should be counselled about the adverse effects of low weight on the skeleton.[23]

In a statement from Massachusetts General Hospital, Dr Anne Klibanski, one of the principal researchers, says, 'Some of these young women are experiencing bone loss comparable to that of women many decades older, despite estrogen therapy. Given this severity and the prevalence of bone loss, the importance of screening all women with anorexia for osteoporosis cannot be over-emphasised.'

Other causes

Cystic fibrosis and inflammatory bowel disease are examples of conditions associated with malabsorption and resultant low bone density in some individuals. The osteoporosis of cystic fibrosis is also related to the frequent need for corticosteroids as well as to other undefined factors.

Drugs

The list of drugs which cause bone loss is extensive and includes, amongst others, glucocorticoids, thyroid hormone (excess), alcohol, medroxyprogesterone acetate (depo provera), luteinizing hormone-releasing hormone agonists, anti-seizure medications, cyclosporine A, aluminium, lithium, and exchange resins.[24]

Glucocorticoids (corticosteroids)

Glucocorticoid use promotes the most common form of drug-related osteoporosis; glucocorticoids are widely used for long-term disorders such as rheumatoid arthritis and other connective tissue diseases, asthma, psoriasis, Crohn's disease, lung disease, inflammatory bowel diseases, severe allergic reactions and inflammations, obstructive pulmonary disease, and in organ transplants. Corticosteroid treatment causes bone loss by a variety of complex mechanisms. It has been shown that bone mineral loss at the hip averages 14 percent in the first year after starting corticosteroid therapy. This is associated with a high rate of fracture — up to *fifty percent* of patients using the drug may fracture, especially post-menopausal women.[25]

Patients treated with 10 mg of the corticosteroid Prednisone for just 20 weeks experienced an eight percent loss of BMD in the spine. High dose treatment (greater than the average daily dose of 7.5 mg Prednisone) has been shown to increase a patient's risk of developing vertebral fractures more than fourfold and doubled their risk of experiencing a hip fracture. Investigators found that even lower daily doses of corticosteroids (between 2.5 mg and 7.5 mg) significantly increased the risk of vertebral fractures by two-and-one-half times. In addition, these lower dose levels increased a patient's risk of developing a hip fracture by more than 75 percent.[26]

Some experts suggest that any patient who receives orally administered glucocorticoids (such as Prednisone or cortisol) in a dose of 5 mg or more for longer than two months is at high risk for excessive bone loss. People who have undergone organ transplant are at high risk for osteoporosis due to a variety of factors, including pre-transplant organ failure and use of glucocorticoids after transplantation.

At this point, the long-term effects on bone of intermittent use of systemic steroids or the chronic use of inhaled steroids, as are often prescribed in asthma, are not known.[27]

Thyroid hormone (L-Thyroxine) replacement therapy
Several studies have shown that long-term thyroxine therapy or high doses of the treatment given to women with hypothyroidism may decrease bone density, particularly in post-menopausal women.[28]

Depo-provera (Medroxyprogesterone Acetate)
This is the contraceptive injection usually given 3-monthly and

also commonly used to treat premenstrual syndrome (PMS), pelvic pain syndrome, endometriosis, and advanced breast cancer in premenopausal women. It has been found to reduce bone density in young women by up to 4.1 percent per year, although bone density increases again once the treatment is stopped. Concerns have been raised about women using the drug around menopause when bone density is naturally decreasing and is unlikely to recover in the way that it does in a younger person when the treatment stops.[29]

Heparin

Continued heparin (blood-thinning) therapy using high doses of the drug is associated with reduced bone density and osteoporosis-related fracture. Warfarin on the other hand has not been reported to have these effects.[30]

Antacids

Continued use of large doses of antacids can cause severe bone pain, rickets (osteomalacia), and fractures. Stopping the treatment will rapidly improve symptoms.

Other drugs

Other drugs which bring about bone loss include anti-convulsants, lithium, neuroleptics used to treat schizophrenia, methotrexate, aluminium, fluoride, exchange resins, and luteinizing hormone-releasing hormone agonists.[31]

Environmental influences

DDT

There is preliminary evidence from two recent studies — one from Sweden and one from Australia — that exposure to the banned pesticide DDT may affect bone mineral density and possibly increase the risk for fragility fractures. In the body,

DDT metabolises into DDE which is known to affect human hormones. A small study of 90 women aged 45 to 65 in northern New South Wales found that those with traces of pesticide in their blood had lower bone density than those with none.[32] A group of 115 men from the general Swedish population and ranging in ages from 40–75 years were similarly tested and a weak association was found between DDE levels and low bone density.[33]

Because DDT was used widely as a pesticide from the 1950s to the 1970s, these groups of women and men could have been exposed to it at the time when spraying was at its peak, and when peak bone mass was being achieved. DDT has a long half-life in the body — about 72 years — so traces are still detectable, even though spraying is no longer permitted in these countries.

Both of these studies were prompted by research two decades ago which showed that DDT affected the fertility of birds and made their eggshells lighter.[34]

Although two initial studies call for larger studies to confirm their findings, they are another salutary reminder of the influence that hormone-mimicking environmental chemicals (organochlorines) may be having on our health. Organochlorines are created by motor vehicle emissions, industrial processes and wastes, and pesticides and herbicides found in waterways, soils and in food. Our bodies are under constant assault from the resulting free radicals (unstable oxygen molecules) which damage our cells and are believed to be at the basis of many 21st century diseases. Since 1980 the incidence of cancer alone has increased by 50 percent in industrialised countries, and from one person in ten in 1950 to one person in three in 2000. It is believed to be linked to avoidable exposures to carcinogens in consumer products, in the air, in water or the workplace.[35]

Some of this damage can be averted through the powerful neutralising effects of naturally occurring dietary antioxidants or free-radical scavengers in fresh fruits and vegetables, and a supplementation with vitamins C and E. The consumption of organic foods and avoidance of exposure to chemicals is fundamental to reducing our risks of disease from a toxic environment.

Consumption of carbonated drinks

A recent US study found that girls who drank carbonated beverages had about three times greater risk of fracture than that of girls who did not drink carbonated beverages. It is likely that the phosphorus contained in soft drinks may damage bone due to the change in the phosphorus-calcium ratio or through increased bone resorption.[36]

Stress and osteoporosis

Stress is generated by the tensions and pressures of work and home life and the constant shortage of time most people live with. We face traffic stress, daily doses of stressful news broadcasts, ever-present crime. All of this stress is metabolised by the body. We have developed a society which makes us sick. Ultimately stress wears the immune system down and eventually chronic untreated stress can make you ill.

Levels of the stress hormone cortisol produced by the adrenal glands rise when we are under stress, then fall when the stress disappears. But chronic stress, a common phenomenon in western life, can override our body's natural ability to bounce back. Sustained stress keeps cortisol levels high, which in turn suppresses our immune response.

If we continue to live in stressful circumstances, we are more likely to develop numerous disorders including infections, obesity, poor wound healing, decreased learning and memory skills, hypertension, stroke, heart attacks and even osteoporosis (low BMD).

High levels of cortisol can result in the extraction of calcium from our bones, and its circulation back into the bloodstream. This means that an excess of cortisol will cause bone loss and ultimately could cause fragile bones. Cortisol can directly suppress DHEA and progesterone. It can also suppress thyroid activity. This means that the conditions and symptoms associated with low DHEA, low progesterone or low thyroid can be caused by high cortisol levels which are linked back to the stress in our lives.

Magnesium deficiency could also be a result of stress, and magnesium is essential for normal bone metabolism. Adrenaline, which is also released by the adrenal glands when we are stressed, draws magnesium out of the cells allowing it to be flushed out in the urine.[37]

It is generally accepted that overall good health is dependent on managing stress. Regular daily exercise, a positive workplace, good friendships and a spiritual dimension to life are said to be helpful. Practice of meditation is also known to reduce stress levels and improve health and wellbeing. In a large study published in the *Journal of Clinical Psychology*, nearly two decades of stress-related studies and various meditation and relaxation techniques were compared statistically. In the results of all the tests together, Transcendental Meditation (TM) was shown to reduce anxiety twice as much as any other technique.[38]

Inadequate nutrition

Nutrition is one of the most important factors to influence bone health and hip fracture risk, but the majority of studies investigate only selected aspects of nutrition — specifically calcium — in relation to osteoporosis. Several studies have noted that elderly patients with hip fractures are likely to have poorer nutritional status when they are admitted to hospital. Sadly, many elderly people fail to receive adequate intakes of most nutrients. It appears that malnutrition is much worse in those who suffer hip fractures. A study of 2,500 white women showed that those who had poor nutrition had a significantly higher rate of hip fracture.[39]

Smoking

Smoking is bad for your bones as well as for your heart and lungs. Women who smoke have lower levels of oestrogen compared to nonsmokers and frequently go through menopause earlier. Postmenopausal women who smoke may require higher doses of hormone replacement therapy and therefore are at risk for more side-effects. Smokers also may absorb less calcium from their diets.[40]

A study of 300 healthy young women aged 20–29 found that smokers had significantly lower spine BMD and a tendency for lower BMD at other sites.[41] According to a recent report, postmenopausal women who smoke cigarettes are significantly more likely to sustain a hip fracture than those who don't smoke.[42]

Alcohol

Alcohol has been linked to reduced bone mass because it disrupts the absorption of calcium. The effect is believed to be significant at levels of more than two drinks per day of spirits, beer, or wine. Chronic alcoholism, particularly in men, significantly increases osteoporosis and fractures of the rib, hip and spine.[43]

However, a recent report from a large French study involving 7,500 women over the age of 75 years found that drinking one to three glasses of wine each day may have a positive effect on bone mass. The authors caution that nutritional and physical exercise factors were likely to be involved in the outcome of their study, so the results couldn't be entirely attributed to the alcohol.[44]

Childhood risk

Children have always fractured their bones and far more fractures occur in this age group than any other because of higher levels of physical activity, risk-taking and so on. Even so, racial factors do seem to play a part. Children of African descent have been found to have denser bone and fewer fractures than white American children.[45] A New Zealand study found that forearm fractures were more common in girls with low bone density throughout the skeleton, and concludes that low BMD may contribute to fracture risk in childhood.[46] The authors conclude that whether this points to fragile bones as an adult has yet to be determined.

DXA scanning is not necessarily accurate in measuring bone density in children. Authors of a recent article warned that 'accurate interpretation of DXA data in children requires consideration of bone size, pubertal stage, skeletal maturation, ethnicity and body composition. Bone mineral content may be underestimated in smaller children and overestimated in larger ones. DXA is a valuable tool for assessing pediatric bone health, but accurate interpretation of densitometry results requires recognition of a myriad of pitfalls.'[47]

Conclusion

Osteoporosis is multifactorial. A diagnosis of low bone density may serve as a warning that some other disorder is behind it. It is therefore extremely important that all possible causes are investigated. Many of the risk factors can be eliminated through lifestyle adjustments, weight-bearing exercise, an appropriate diet and the avoidance of falls. Others can be managed by a conscientious doctor who identifies a medical risk factor and treats it with an awareness of possible consequences to bone.

There are a variety of tests to determine risks for secondary causes. See Appendix II on page 206 for more information.

CHAPTER SIX

Treatments for osteoporosis
– introduction

THE REDEFINING OF OSTEOPOROSIS AS A MEASURE OF low bone density has been discussed in previous chapters. Bone density is only one aspect of bone health. It doesn't tell us anything about the micro-structure or strength of our bones. As we have seen, low bone mineral density can be normal for many people. One of the difficulties in presenting the available evidence for the treatment of fragile bones is that most often studies are measuring changes in bone density — that is, how much bone density loss has been slowed down, or even some cases where bone density has increased. There are few studies that measure a reduction in fragility fractures. In most cases, treatments are treating a risk factor, not the established disease.

There is not a single pharmaceutical treatment known to actually reverse osteoporosis by repairing and rebuilding damaged or fragile bone. Drugs that can increase bone density are not able to reverse the loss of bone strength that occurs in severe osteoporosis when the trabecular struts are severed. No bone agent is able to rebuild severed connections.[1]

Treatments for low bone density can be grouped into two main categories — those that decrease bone resorption, the dissolving of old bone; and those that increase bone formation, the building of new bone. Most of the treatments currently used are the former, anti-resorptive drugs. HRT is anti-resorptive medication. Bisphosphonates are also anti-resorptive. There is no clinical treatment at this time that can both decrease bone resorption and maintain a relatively high level of bone formation.

More than ten years ago studies were done to measure the effect of sodium fluoride on bone. Fluoride was well known for its ability to increase bone mineral density and many felt that long-term studies of its effect on fractures were not necessary. However, the studies found that although fluoride brought about huge increases in spinal bone mineral density it didn't reduce the incidence of fractures. In fact, fractures were found to be *higher* in the fluoride group than in the placebo group. Apparently the new bone was of poor quality.[2] Therefore even a treatment that increases bone formation and improves bone density may not result in a dramatic improvement in fracture outcomes. This study also further confirms that bone density testing is not a good method of predicting fracture.

Current drug treatments could be dangerous for users. It is possible that truly safe and effective treatments will emerge in the future, but at this time it appears they are only able to slow down bone density loss, with the potential of a heavy price to pay. Given that low bone density is only one of many risk factors, and not a good predictor of future fracture, it may be better to avoid drugs altogether in preference for lifestyle changes known to influence bone health and overall health.

The popular idea that calcium tablets or the daily glass of milk will keep bones strong remains unsubstantiated. An adequate intake of foods high in all bone nutrients — calcium, magnesium, potassium, and other essential vitamins and minerals including vitamin D — is fundamental. Minimising calcium loss through a healthy diet rich in fruit and vegetables and low in meat protein and other acid-forming foods is also recommended, as are managing stress, not smoking and limiting alcohol intake.

Regular exercise is the single most important strategy for bone health. It puts weight on the skeleton and forces muscles to pull against the bones. Exercise, appropriate diet and supplemental bone nutrients are simple steps that may be the most effective treatments for minimising bone loss and preventing fracture.

The following chapters consider the evidence for:

- Medical treatments
- Calcium and dairy consumption
- Nutrition generally
- Exercise.

Note that when a percentage improvement or increased risk from a treatment is identified, it is important to recognise that it represents a percentage of the risk that already exists. For example, a 35 percent reduction in bone loss as a result of a treatment means that if a person already has a three percent risk of bone loss over two years, that risk has been reduced by 35 percent. This would then reduce the risk from three percent to two percent.

CHAPTER SEVEN

Hormone replacement therapy – 'First, do no harm'

M ILLIONS OF BABY-BOOM ERA WOMEN FIND THEM-selves facing the difficult decision of whether or not to take hormone replacement therapy (HRT): either short-term to help them manage the menopause transition, or long-term to protect against osteoporosis. Frequently encouraged by their doctors to embark upon the treatment as a means to replace the now 'missing' reproductive hormones oestrogen and progesterone, they are confused by conflicting reports of its effectiveness and its safety. This can cause considerable anxiety for those who proceed to take it, and further worry for those who don't. Unbiased evidence-based information is difficult to come by.

Forty years ago, the western world thought that medicine had discovered the holy grail in the form of supplemental synthetic oestrogen — a medicine claimed to virtually stop women from ageing. Massive marketing campaigns appealed to women's vanity and desire for 'eternal youth', as well as promising relief from all manner of menopause-related problems. Easily convinced that they were hormone deficient, and that here was a solution, menopausal women in their droves began oestrogen replacement therapy.

But as time went by it became apparent that many of the women using oestrogen were developing endometrial cancer, or cancer of the womb. Normally a rare form of cancer, it was clearly linked to the supplemental hormone. This came as a huge blow for the burgeoning industry and resulted in the withdrawal of the drug and the redevelopment of the combined oestrogen/progestogen (or progestin) regime which more closely mimicked the menstrual cycle. The new combination all but eliminated the endometrial cancer risk.

Back on the market and now called hormone replacement therapy, the treatment's advertised benefits started to read like those of a wonder drug again. It was maintained that HRT would not only relieve hot flushes, it would also, on the basis of scant evidence, keep a woman's skin youthful, restore lost memory, deal to irritability, mood swings, lowered libido, and prevent a raft of serious diseases. Even as recently as 1999, on the cover of the book *The HRT Solution — Restoring Vitality, Sexuality and Health*, the authors claim: 'In addition to recharging your batteries and relieving menopausal symptoms, hormone replacement can help stop bone loss and protect your heart and brain from the degenerative processes commonly associated with ageing.'[1]

HRT use continues to expand globally. But these days, evidence for its effectiveness is severely limited and new evidence for serious risks associated with use continues to frighten women and batter the industry.

HRT's benefits at menopause have been reduced to the

relief of hot flushes and vaginal dryness.[2] Its application as a treatment for women with established heart disease has now been dismissed. Earlier studies which showed a reduced risk of cardiovascular disease in HRT users (and resulted in widespread prescribing) were finally deemed flawed because their results were due to the selection of healthy women who were unlikely to develop symptoms anyway.[3] A large four-year clinical trial in women with established heart disease showed no benefit overall, and worryingly, a significantly higher incidence of fatal heart attack in the first year of use. It also showed a three-fold increased risk for blood clots in the legs or deep venous thrombosis (DVT) in the HRT group. As a consequence, and pending further evidence, it is no longer recommended as a treatment for heart disease, although many women continue to take it for this purpose.[4]

Evidence that long-term use of HRT (more than five years) is associated with an increased risk for breast cancer is now substantial — particularly in women who take combined oestrogen and progestogen, and are of lean build.[5] Although the increased risk is deemed to be small, it becomes greater the longer HRT is taken, and the older a woman becomes.[6]

Neither has the hoped-for evidence emerged that HRT protects against Alzheimer's disease, nor helps with mental clarity, mood swings or depression.[7]

That leaves osteoporosis. The promoters of HRT emphasise its long-term application for the prevention of osteoporosis, but a serious look at the evidence reveals that the benefits in terms of fracture prevention are virtually nonexistent. With the known risks associated with long-term use it is surprising that its prescription for osteoporosis can be justified at all.

Two very large randomised controlled trials, WHI (Women's

Health Initiative) and WISDOM (Women's International Study of Long Duration after Menopause), are currently underway to measure the benefits and risks from long-term use of HRT by healthy women. Those results are expected sometime between 2005 and 2010, but preliminary results from the WHI trial involving 27,000 US women indicate a higher level of heart attack, stroke, and blood clots in the legs and lungs (as well as deaths caused by them) in the HRT group in the first two years of use.[8] This is the first evidence of risk associated with short-term use of HRT by well women, and raises serious questions about the ethics of prescribing HRT under any circumstances until safety is assured.

HRT market continues to grow

Despite the now huge credibility gap in the industry, the HRT market continues to expand globally with the current US$3 billion of sales expected to at least double in the next five years.[9] Powerful commercial interests continue to place heavy and continuing pressure on policymakers, doctors and patients to adopt the bone density screening/HRT solution to osteoporosis. Each year doctors prescribe HRT to millions of women and today about one third of all US women aged 45 to 65 (some 16 million) are using it.[10] New Zealand with its much smaller population of 3.8 million has 100,000 women currently using HRT.

So embedded is the belief that women will benefit from such a strategy that resisting it can be made incredibly difficult for the patient who dares.

When Irene's bone densitometry test gave her a diagnosis of osteopenia (low bone mass), she was determined to manage the matter herself, to research it thoroughly, and embark on a proactive programme of exercise and dietary changes. She felt well, had never fractured, had no family history of osteoporosis, and wanted to take responsibility for the situation. Besides, she was wary of taking HRT long term as she was very conscious of the controversy surrounding the drug. But her doctor was unhappy with her decision and insisted that she was at serious risk for debilitating fracture unless she complied. Her refusal set off an astonishing chain of events involving formal letters and phone calls from the doctor, and enormous emotional pressure, which although unsuccessful in altering her decision, ultimately caused Irene huge anxiety, and served to greatly exaggerate the seriousness of her condition.

Irene's situation is not unique. Women frequently comment on the non-negotiable attitude of the medical profession when it comes to the management of their low bone density. The diagnosis and the treatment have become inseparable in the minds of many doctors. The model which advocates the medical management of bone and bone health across a person's lifespan has become institutionalised in a matter of a very few years.

Unfortunately this draws attention away from the important problems of diet, exercise, lifestyle, and the identification of other osteoporosis risk factors such as prescribed drug use, alcohol abuse, eating disorders in young women, poverty, unsafe environments for the elderly, malnutrition, and so on.

Menopause and fracture — is there a link?

A vast medical paradigm has developed around the concept of the 'oestrogen-deficient woman', based on the questionable theory that once a woman is postmenopausal she is in a hormonally deficient state requiring regular fixed doses of synthetic hormones to bring her back to 'normal' and to protect her bones.

Women are not hormone-deficient after menopause. The ovaries go on producing lesser amounts of oestrogen and the body achieves a new stable balance of hormones, including lower levels of oestrogen and more male-type androgens. Directly contradicting popular understanding, a recent study published in the *New England Journal of Medicine* indicated that the majority of women over 65 produce enough oestrogen naturally to give them bone protection, raising further serious questions about whether HRT has a role in women's health at all.[11]

Whether altered or lowered levels of hormones cause fragility fractures is questionable. When the hormone levels of postmenopausal Mayan women of Central America were measured they were found to have oestrogen levels no higher than those of white American women — even lower in some cases. They live for an average of 30 years after menopause and they don't lose height, don't develop a dowager's hump, and don't get fractures. Bone density tests showed that they lost bone density at the same rate as US women.[12]

If osteoporosis-related fractures are due to oestrogen deficiency it would be reasonable to expect that women with the disease have lower levels of oestrogen than women without the disorder. This is not the case. Studies have found that oestrogen levels are similar in postmenopausal women with and without osteoporosis.[13]

The argument weakens further when you consider that ALL women go through menopause, but not all women are at risk for fracture. African-American women, for example, have a twofold lower risk of fracture, and in countries like Ghana, Guinea and the Congo, osteoporosis is extremely rare. Asian women have lower rates of fracture and Hispanic women have approximately half as many fractures as Caucasian women.

Do all women lose bone at menopause?

Thinning of bones in women as they age has long been blamed on menopause, and in particular the drop in the production of oestrogen by the ovaries at this time. It has been estimated and generally accepted as true that women lose about 12–15 percent of their bone mass in the years immediately after menopause. But it is now known that bone loss around menopause varies hugely from woman to woman. Studies have shown that although some women lose a lot of bone density quickly around the years after menopause, others lose comparatively little, or even none at all.[14]

A recent analysis of bone density in an HRT and non-HRT treated (placebo) group of 701 postmenopausal women aged 64 years and under, showed that about half of the women in the placebo group did not appear to lose bone density in the three years they were studied.[15]

In 1995 the US Congress Office of Technology Assessment reported on their comprehensive systematic review of the evidence on bone mass loss at menopause. The review concludes that the evidence does not support the widely held hypothesis that the rate of bone loss is greatly accelerated immediately following menopause.[16]

The association of menopause and bone loss could in fact come from the fact that many bone studies have been done on women whose ovaries were removed, not those who underwent a normal menopause. Surgical menopause seems to accelerate bone loss. A woman who has had her ovaries removed has double the loss of bone compared to a woman going through a natural menopause.[17]

HRT and menopause

Women are often exhorted to take HRT to mask the symptoms of menopause as they negotiate the sometimes rocky transition from their fertile years. Many have been led to believe it will stave off the ageing process, keep them 'sane', and eliminate unpleasant symptoms like mood swings, anxiety, irritability, memory loss and fatigue. But HRT has been shown to be effective only in treating hot flushes and night sweats, and in a localised form, vaginal dryness.[18] Despite this, many doctors routinely prescribe it as the panacea for all the mostly minor irritations of menopause in the misguided belief that it is beneficial.

It is not just the doctors. A whole sub-set of midlife women subscribe to the theory that HRT is essential — the popular rationale being that it keeps a woman young and prevents a host of diseases associated with ageing. It is a powerful justification which can put pressure on other women and also doctors who may be reluctant to prescribe. Researchers in Sheffield, England, questioned new HRT users and found that although women were worried about the breast cancer risk, most of them would use HRT if they received 'proper counselling'. Forty-four percent of the women expected HRT to make them 'feel new' and 18 percent thought it would make them stay young.[19]

HRT comes in different forms — pills, patches, creams and rings, and many different brands. Some types of HRT are labelled 'natural' because they are made from horses' oestrogen or synthesised in a laboratory from soy isoflavones. Different regimes and doses have different effects, and debate continues about the optimum dose for older women at risk for osteoporosis.

Side-effects of HRT

Side-effects range from headaches, breast tenderness, leg cramps and bloating to the more serious break-through bleeding and build up of abnormal (pre-cancerous) tissue in the womb lining. For many women the side-effects are intolerable, and are the reason they discontinue using HRT. Suddenly introducing fixed doses of synthetic ovarian hormones into the body of a woman who has long since ceased menstruating is very likely to result in problems. Even younger women can find it uncomfortable.

> Kate went through menopause early — in her late thirties. She had troublesome hot flushes and fluctuating energy levels. Her doctor prescribed HRT, believing this would help. And it did, for a while. But gradually Kate developed migraine headaches of such intensity that some days she couldn't function at all. As they became more frequent, and altered doses of HRT made little difference, she decided to stop the treatment. But instead of gradually reducing the dose, she stopped abruptly. The physiological reaction was dramatic — equivalent to an instant menopause. Her hot flushes returned with such intensity that it was necessary to go back on HRT, endure more headaches and gradually ease off before she could feel normal again.

HRT reduces bone loss

Evidence that oestrogen replacement could slow down postmenopausal bone loss provided a whole new direction for drug companies when the hormone's link to endometrial cancer made its use increasingly controversial. Once it reappeared on the market as the new combined HRT and the endometrial cancer risk was reduced, it became the gold standard treatment for osteoporosis. These days it has increasing competition from the bisphosphonate Alendronate (Fosamax).

HRT is known to slow down bone density loss in most postmenopausal women who use it, and even to slightly increase bone density in some cases. This effect is not observed in all women who take HRT however, and it has been noted that those who smoke or who have low body weight particularly are less likely to respond to HRT.[20, 21]

The fact that it slows bone density loss is the point upon which the entire industry pivots. If it can slow down bone density loss, then it can 'prevent' osteoporosis. That is assuming a definition of osteoporosis as a measure of low bone density. Increasing bone density through drug therapy, and actually preventing fractures, are two very different goals in managing osteoporosis, but one is very often confused with the other. The real question has to be, does HRT prevent fracture in those who have used it?

Many experts now agree that it is probably useless and potentially dangerous to take a drug at menopause in the hope of preventing fractures which may occur decades later. Because of the risks associated with long-term use of HRT, current recommendations are that women start treatment later, maybe in their sixties when they are considered more at risk for fracture. But this would still require long-term treatment —

ten, twenty years — to offer possible bone protection in later years.

A recent report on how many older women continue to take HRT indicated that they may not be using the treatment long enough to benefit from its predicted effects. The authors of the report point out that HRT must be used consistently for at least four years in order to gain any benefit. Yet only 20 percent of older women who start HRT continue treatment for at least this long.[22] The reasons for giving up are most often due to side-effects. Older women can experience break-through menstrual bleeding, breast tenderness and headaches. Careful management of dosage may help alleviate these problems, but they contribute to the reluctance many feel to take HRT.

> Alice is one such case. At the age of 75 she was pre-scribed HRT because the bone density in her hip is -3 SDs below the young norm, well below the level which the WHO defines as osteoporosis. She is a small person, very active and well, with no previous fractures. As soon as she began to take the hormones her breasts became tender, then gradually so sore that she couldn't touch them. She started menstruating again, even though the form of HRT she was taking was supposed to eliminate that possibility. Such was the degree of discomfort experienced, Alice elected to come off HRT and reconsider her options.

Generally compliance, or continuation of therapy, is poor. Studies indicate that 20–30 percent of women who are given prescriptions for HRT fail to have them filled, and for those who do, the continuation after eight to twelve months is only 30–40 percent.[23]

The waning effect of HRT

Studies also show that any protective effect from reducing bone turnover and slowing bone density loss is sustained only as long as the treatment is taken. There is also an acknowledged 'waning effect' in older women. *In women aged 75 years or more, the group most at risk for fracture, it has been observed that there is little difference in bone density between those who have taken HRT long term, and those who have not.*[24] In addition, once the treatment is stopped, the loss accelerates again, regardless of how long HRT has been taken, and bone density after ten years is similar to that of those who have never taken hormones. This has led many doctors to conclude that in order to have any benefit, the drugs should be taken for life. Unfortunately, long-term use of HRT may increase the risk for breast cancer in particular, as we shall see in the next section.

HRT — the risks

Breast cancer

Despite a lack of evidence from large placebo-controlled trials, most researchers agree that there is a small but substantial risk of breast cancer with longer-term use of HRT. A recent updated report from the landmark Nurses' Health Study showed that after five years' use of HRT the annual increased risk was 9 percent for combined HRT and 3.3 percent for oestrogen alone.* [25]

An analysis of 51 studies showed that women who have used HRT for more than 11 years have a 35 percent increased risk of breast cancer compared to women who have never used HRT. The risk becomes greater with age and length of use, and disappears five years after HRT is discontinued.[26]

---

* These figures represent a percentage of the existing risk (see page 109).

A Swedish study also found greater risks with combined HRT; for six or more years of current or recent use the risk of breast cancer was increased by 70 percent for combined therapy but no increase was seen for oestrogen alone.[27]

The most recent large study followed 46,000 women for ten years to see whether the adding of progestogen to the HRT regimen increased breast cancer risk. The study concluded that the postmenopausal use of oestrogen therapy, when it includes progestogen, significantly increases the risk that a woman will develop breast cancer by age 70 years, particularly smaller lean women. The authors concluded that each year of use of HRT increased the risk of breast cancer by 8 percent. The combined therapy was more risky than oestrogen alone.[28] In this, the largest study completed to date measuring the risks of breast cancer, researchers found there was nearly double the risk of breast cancer if women continue HRT for over a decade. The high risk disappeared within four years of stopping HRT.[29]

An accompanying editorial in the *Journal of the American Medical Association* in 2000 warns: '. . . the risks and benefits of prolonged use of postmenopausal hormones should be re-examined in the light of a likely substantial increase in risk of breast cancer with combined therapy.' And concludes: 'The commonly held belief that ageing routinely requires pharmacological management has unfortunately led to neglect of diet and lifestyle as the primary means to achieve healthy ageing. Now is an appropriate time to reassess this emphasis.'[29]

HRT has been conservatively estimated to cause an excess of 2, 6, and 12 breast cancers for every 1,000 women who use it for 5, 10, and 15 years respectively.[30]

Women are offered the reassurance that it is not believed to increase deaths from breast cancer when treated women are regularly screened and breast cancers are diagnosed early as a result. But there is the added problem that HRT alters breast tissue density and is associated with a higher rate of wrong diagnoses — both negative and positive. A recent Australian study found that the sensitivity of mammography at detecting cancer has been found to be significantly lower in HRT users, especially in women aged 50–69 years.[31]

Modest alcohol consumption and HRT use is also associated with an increased risk of breast cancer.[32]

Ovarian cancer

A recent large study of 46,260 postmenopausal women, which looked at the number of deaths from ovarian cancer in those taking oestrogen alone, found that more than ten years' use was associated with an increased risk of ovarian cancer that persisted up to 29 years after cessation of use.[33] The risk of ovarian cancer was approximately doubled in women who had used oestrogen for ten or more years, but was not evident in less than ten years of use. The impact of HRT — combined oestrogen and progestogen — on ovarian cancer risk is unknown.

Endometrial cancer

For users of oestrogen replacement alone there is a three- to fivefold increased risk for endometrial cancer (cancer of the lining of the womb) but this risk is averted by the addition of progestogen to the HRT regime in women with an intact uterus.[34] Unfortunately this combination has now been linked to a greater risk for breast cancer.

Heart attack and stroke

A large four-year placebo-controlled trial which showed no benefit overall from HRT to women with established risk factors for heart disease, did however show a significantly higher incidence of fatal heart attack in the first year of use, along with increased deep venous thrombosis, pulmonary embolism (leg and lung clots) and gallbladder disease in the HRT group.[35]

Twenty years of follow-up in the Nurses' Health Study shows that daily higher oestrogen doses of 0.625 mg or higher along with progestogen may increase the risk of stroke by up to 45 percent.[36] An accompanying editorial recommends 'that clinicians should not use hormone replacement therapy for prevention of coronary disease until this practice is supported by evidence from randomised trials'.[37]

As previously discussed, preliminary results recently released from the large US government Women's Health Initiative (WHI) 11-year trial involving 27,000 women aged 50–79 indicate that healthy women *without* established risk factors for heart disease using HRT had experienced more heart attacks, strokes, deep vein thrombosis and pulmonary embolism (leg and lung clots) than controls *in the first two years* of the study.[38] This alarming and surprising outcome adds to the evidence that HRT does not protect against cardiovascular problems, and even worse, may cause them. Most importantly, this appears to be the first serious negative finding from the *short-term* use of HRT. It has previously been believed that short-term use is safe, and it has been long-term use that has linked HRT to an increased risk for breast cancer.

On the recommendation of the US Data and Safety Monitoring Board every woman in the trial was informed by letter in April 2000 of the adverse findings which had affected around 1 percent of the participants overall. They were also advised that the board, which had met twice to examine the findings and decide whether to halt the study, had recommended that the 11-year WHI trial continue. The 27,000 women were told 'Your safety is our first concern . . . Your continued participation in the WHI program is now more important than ever. This new information highlights the critical role you play in finding answers to questions about hormones and women's health . . . We thank you once again for helping us find answers for generations of women to come!'[39] It is reported that very few women left the trial after receiving the letter.

Other than a general press release at the time and the letter sent to the trial participants, the data from the WHI trial remains protected and the actual information has not been released for view. Editorial in a major medical journal commented recently: 'These findings are preliminary but they would not have been released in this manner if they were not substantial. Hormone therapy appears to be having the same initial effect on coronary risk among healthy women as among women . . . with documented coronary disease.'[40] Final results from the WHI will not be available until 2005, and clinicians have meantime been advised to not change their practice.

A finding such as this highlights again the fact that many questions about the safety of HRT remain unanswered. Given that current evidence indicates HRT only really benefits the woman who has severe hot flushes and vaginal dryness (for which there are effective alternative treatments), and that it has not been proven to offer any other benefit, the preliminary findings from the WHI trial must raise questions about the ethics of prescribing it at all. If an early increased risk could be death and serious disease, surely HRT should only be offered when the risk to not offer it leads to a similar risk of death and serious disease? This new information demands a total reassessment of the risks and benefits of offering HRT to healthy women.

Other risks

HRT causes a small increased risk of gallstone formation. Women who use HRT also have a twofold increased risk of developing lupus erythematosus.[41] Because of the threefold increased blood-clotting risk it is recommended that HRT be withheld for 90 days after any surgery.[42] Recent analysis of data from the Nurses' Health Study indicated that women using oestrogen alone or combined HRT had a greater risk of asthma than women not taking hormones.[43]

HRT and fracture protection

Many doctors agree that it is probably of little value to take a drug at age 50 in the hope of preventing fractures decades later. In fact it is potentially dangerous. Women could be trading a possible wrist fracture in their 70s for breast cancer.

Fracture as result of fragile bones is what correctly defines established osteoporosis. For this reason it is supremely important for any treatment regime to have strong evidence that it will prevent fractures, not just influence bone density. Currently there is no evidence from randomised controlled trials that HRT prevents fracture in women with low spinal bone density, or that it prevents fractures in older women or fractures of the hip. There is limited and debatable evidence that HRT protects against fracture of the vertebrae in women with pre-existing fractures.

To date, the evidence for the anti-fracture effect of HRT comes primarily from observational studies, which are generally considered less reliable. Early observational studies indicated a reduction in hip fractures in women taking HRT, but the limitation of the studies was that they were generally based on comparatively young women (mostly under 75) who were less likely to fracture at that age. The studies also showed that any protection possibly offered by HRT was lost within a few years after stopping hormone replacement therapy.[44]

The most significant evidence available at this point comes from the large four-year randomised clinical trial of 2,763 women of average age 66.7 years with pre-existing cardio-vascular disease. After four years the HRT users did *not* show any anti-fracture benefit.[45]

There is weak evidence that HRT will reduce fractures in healthy younger postmenopausal women. One recent trial of 368 women showed a small reduction in non-vertebral fractures in women who were early postmenopausal.[46] A closer look at the study raises questions. These women had no risk factors for osteoporosis and sustained a total of 39 fractures over five years including ankle, foot and even skull — fractures which are not associated with osteoporosis. Unlike most studies which focus on low-impact fractures, this one included all high-energy fractures including bicycle accidents. In the HRT group, 7.5 percent of the women fractured, and in the placebo group 12 percent fractured. The authors reported that the results were *not* statistically significant, until they made some adjustments after the initial analysis. A post-hoc analysis is generally not considered to be good science. This study was funded by the HRT-producing drug company, Schering.

One other possibly relevant study, a very small randomised

controlled trial, measured the effect of HRT on 75 post-menopausal women with one or more existing vertebral fractures due to osteoporosis. Thirty-nine of the women received HRT and 39 women received a placebo for one year.[47] During that time seven women had eight new vertebral fractures in the HRT group and 12 women had a total of 20 new vertebral fractures in the placebo group. That is, several women had more than one fracture. Fractures in the spine are considered to be interrelated events, so the number of women fracturing is more significant than the number of fractures. This interpretation renders the outcome insignificant.[48] This study was also funded by a drug company.

There are alternatives

Pharmaceuticals like HRT have been popularised as the solution to low bone density, even though substantial evidence exists that weight-bearing exercise can also alter and improve bone density, while offering other major health benefits.[49] Adequate bone nutrients and a diet rich in fruit, vegetables and plant protein are safe and effective alternatives for well women. A recent report from Asia confirming that soy products are protective against bone loss in Chinese women concludes that many are considering soy as an alternative to hormone replacement therapy. Very few Asian women choose to use HRT. For example, only 2.9 percent of women aged 53 to 55 years use hormone replacement therapy in Hong Kong.[50]

Neither is HRT the only option a woman has for treating her hot flushes. There is evidence from randomised trials that black cohosh (*Cimicifuga racemosa*) relieves hot flushes as effectively as HRT without the risks or side-effects.[51] For the last 40 years women in Germany with hot flushes are more likely to be recommended to use black cohosh than HRT by their doctors.

Could HRT cause bone nutrient deficiencies?

An article published in the *Journal of Nutritional and Environmental Medicine* in 1998 challenges current beliefs that osteoporosis is due to deficiencies of calcium and oestrogen, and suggests that it is due to nutritional deficiencies linked to synthetic hormone use.[52] It questions the effectiveness of HRT, saying that in spite of numerous publications claiming short-term benefits, there is also substantial published evidence to show that women taking hormones are more likely to have nutrient deficiencies and imbalances than women not taking hormones. Women who take hormones have been found to have significantly lower levels of white cell zinc, lower red cell magnesium, and abnormally high serum copper levels. These nutrient imbalances are likely to impair normal bone formation as studies of HRT users observed significantly lower levels of the bone enzyme alkaline phosphatase (ALP) — the enzyme which is an indicator of how much bone rebuilding is occurring.

The authors conclude that it is ironic that hormone taking — in the form of the oral contraceptive or HRT — in developed countries could be contributing to the higher rates of osteoporosis-related fracture observed in those countries.

Is our safety being compromised?

We have seen that the WHO definition based on bone density bears little relationship to osteoporosis as defined by bone fragility. In just twenty years a disease has quite simply been created by a change in definition; a reason for the disease has been found in the form of menopause; and a drug is conveniently available to treat the disease.

Besieged by frightening statistics, messages from the media, and flyers in doctors' waiting rooms and in pharmacies, women have been convinced that menopause is the primary cause of osteoporosis. But the main cause of bone-density-related osteoporosis is ageing, not menopause. Everyone — men and women — loses bone density as they age, but the rate of loss at menopause varies hugely. Despite substantial evidence to the contrary, and obvious serious risks, many general practitioners remain convinced that menopause, osteoporosis and HRT go together, and that women are to be persuaded of the fact.

Common sense has been abandoned. Few medical practitioners appear to question the appropriateness of prescribing potent medication to women for menopause, which is not a medical condition, not an illness, but a normal life passage. Neither do they question the wisdom of treating healthy women with no symptoms for osteoporosis with a drug which has not been proven to prevent fracture. The greatest concern is that in all the hype and confusion created by drug and device companies pushing products, and advocates seeking to further their causes, millions of women are being wrongly diagnosed and are taking potentially dangerous medications for a disease they do not and will not ever have.

As we go to press:

A meta-analysis of 22 randomised trials of HRT has noted a 35 percent reduction in non-vertebral fractures (hip and wrist) in women under the age of 60 who are using HRT, but no reduction in women over 60 years.[53] The accompanying editorial observes that the anti-fracture evidence is weak due to the poor quality of some of the studies, and that as women in their fifties have a relatively low rate of fracture anyway, the benefits of long-term treatment may not exceed the risks. The US FDA has recently withdrawn its approval of HRT as a treatment for osteoporosis.[54]

CHAPTER EIGHT

Bisphosphonates and other treatments

BISPHOSPHONATES ARE RELATIVELY NEW DRUGS IN THE osteoporosis treatment arsenal and are considered a useful alternative treatment option for women who cannot or prefer not to take hormone replacement. They are also considered appropriate for use by men. But the lack of safety data, and the way that they act on bone by suppressing bone turnover, are causing some experts to advocate caution in their use. They can also have unpleasant side-effects.

Bisphosphonates like Fosamax (also called Alendronate) are non-hormonal drugs approved by the US Food and Drug Administration (FDA) to treat osteoporosis. They are synthetic compounds which bind to bone mineral crystals and inhibit bone resorption. They are known to be effective in slowing bone loss and can even increase spinal density in some cases. A patient gets 'one shot' at the bisphosphonate bone density increasing effect, after which time continued use of the drug only maintains bone density.

There are no long-term studies completed at this time which indicate what the benefits or risks over time may be. Although there is evidence for a reduction in clinical fractures in older women with previous vertebral fractures in the first three years of use, there are now indications that fracture rates may begin to increase again after longer use. Osteoporosis expert Dr Susan Ott commented recently: 'In adult women with osteoporosis the bisphosphonates are effective for 4.5 years, but maybe not longer than that, more data is really needed. Up to 7 years no serious side-effects have been seen, but there might be more vertebral fractures during years 6–7.'[1]

Treatment options for osteoporosis in the young are virtually non-existent, although bisphosphonates are being trialled in some countries. Because bisphosphonates suppress bone remodelling, the potential for these drugs to do harm to the young skeleton has raised concerns about their use.

All bisphosphonates work by inhibiting the action of the osteoclast cells. This slows down bone resorption. In other words, they disrupt the mechanism which allows osteoclasts to remove old weakened bone so that osteoblast cells can build new bone. But osteoblasts require the activity of osteoclasts and the resorption of old bone to trigger their activity. In the absence of osteoclasts, osteoblasts are immobilised. This explains the increase in bone density that occurs in the first year or so of use, but also explains the subsequent plateau, and the lack of evidence for long-term benefits. Bisphosphonate drugs therefore interfere with the process of bone remodelling. In an older person who has too much bone resorption and not enough bone building this may be a good thing on a short-term basis. It allows the old bone to be retained, and in the first three years of use will usually show a modest increase in bone mineral density and possibly some protection against fractures.

However, new bone can only be built after old bone is removed. These drugs halt the bone turnover process and there is now initial evidence that retaining old bone could mean an increase in microfractures and weakness leading to bone fragility. The effect of long-term use of the treatment is not known, as the drugs are still relatively new. Alendronate deposits in the bone for over ten years and will accumulate with use. Just stopping taking the drug will not remove it from the body, and its influence would continue for better or worse. At the same time, short-term use of bisphosphonates is not recommended — i.e. bone returns to the level it was at the start very quickly. Dr Susan Ott cautions: 'I do not think it is wise to give Alendronate for longer than 4.5 years. I would have to see definite proof of safety and benefit to the bones (in terms of fractures) before I would give it longer than that.'[2]

There are concerns that long-term use will produce an older skeleton with more crystallised bone which will have less tensile strength in places like the hip. A recent animal study revealed this to be the case. Bones showed an increase in microdamage (microfracture) and reduced bone toughness after one year of high doses of the bisphosphonates Alendronate (Fosamax) and Risedronate.[3]

Side-effects

Another downside with bisphosphonates is that they can have unpleasant side-effects and present difficulties associated with taking them. It is necessary to accept a strict regime in order to prevent serious stomach problems and maximise absorption. The drugs must be taken on an empty stomach, and without lying down for at least 30 minutes because of the risk of irritating or even make holes in the wall of the oesophagus.

Alendronate may cause problems when combined with other drugs. In a recent study, researchers found that 10 mg a day of Alendronate plus 500 mg of Naproxen (a non-steroidal anti-inflammatory drug) twice a day, produced ulcers in 38 percent of the volunteers and significant side-effects in 69 percent. They conclude that it is clear that Alendronate and Naproxen act synergistically in inducing stomach ulcers.[4]

Other bisphosphonates include Etidronate, Risedronate, Pamidronate, and Ibandronate. Studies with an earlier version of Etidronate showed that it could impair the mineralisation of bone and cause rickets (osteomalacia) when used in a high dose.[5]

The most commonly reported side-effects with Risedronate were back pain, infection, nausea, headache, peripheral oedema, diarrhoea and abdominal pain.

Are the benefits exaggerated?

There is a lot of hype and advertising associated with drugs for osteoporosis. Fosamax is produced by the drug company Merck. One promotional brochure which features four beaming older women in bathing suits and brightly ornamental bathing caps claims: 'Fosamax can help build strong bones which don't fracture so easily.' Another claims: 'A breakthrough that can reverse the progression of osteoporosis at all affected sites.'

It is important to keep in mind that the ads for these medicines typically make them sound more impressive than they actually are. That is because the adverts fail to explain what the stated relative risk or benefit actually means. For example, Fosamax adverts claims a 44 percent reduction in vertebral fractures compared to a placebo. That is sort of true, and it sounds impressive. But the actual or absolute reduction in fractures is only 1.7 percent. In the large definitive Fosamax trial called the Fracture Intervention Trial, 2.1 percent of 2,000 women of average age 68 years taking Fosamax suffered a vertebral fracture, compared with 3.8 percent of 2,000 women who took the placebo. The reduction stated in the advertisement was in fact 44 percent, but of the already small 3.8 percent average fracture rate.[6]

A review of the study concludes that in women with low bone density, 60 of them will need treatment with Fosamax for three years *in order to prevent one fracture* detected on an X-ray. Many consider that this is not sufficient reason to treat, and that the trial really showed no benefit at all. Especially as these are not really vertebral fractures; they are deformities, and typically have no symptoms.[7]

Expert commentary on this study from Dr R. Heaney cautions that the results are minimal and concludes: '. . . with the exception of asymptomatic spine deformities, the anti-fracture benefit of bisphosphonates in women with low bone mass but without prevalent fractures must be judged to be small.'[8] In the same commentary the point is made that although bone density increased in the patients taking Fosamax, it did not make a significant difference to fracture incidence overall which again questions the relevance of bone density as the basis for diagnosing the disease. In other words, if BMD is the main risk factor for osteoporosis, it would be expected that after 4.5 years of increased BMD there would be a noticeable reduction in fractures. Dr Heaney also points out that this raises a dilemma for the conscientious doctor whose patient has been identified with low bone density, but does not have a history of fracture.

There were two arms to the Fracture Intervention Trial: 2,000 women who already had vertebral compression fractures and 4,000 women (already mentioned) who did not. The women all had bone density at the hip that was lower than the average value for a 65-year-old woman. The women in the group of 2000 had low bone mass and previous vertebral fractures — a less common condition that is known to pose a higher risk of further fracturing. After three years of taking Fosamax, these women had fewer new spinal deformities or fractures (8 percent in the Fosamax group compared with 15 percent in the placebo group) as well as 4.6 percent fewer other clinical fractures. Interpretation of the results concludes that twenty-two women need to be treated with Fosamax for three years in order to prevent one vertebral fracture.[9] All treated women in the trial had an increase in bone density.

This double-armed 'definitive' trial was funded by Merck, the producers of Fosamax. Drafts of the study were reviewed, and changes were made by staff at Merck and the co-authors. Three of the main authors declare that they have been in the pay of the company, as speakers in conferences. Since the release of this study, sales of Fosamax have skyrocketed, reaching US$1 billion in 1999. And it hasn't stopped there. From the Merck 2001 financial report: 'Fosamax, the leading nonhormonal product worldwide for the treatment of osteoporosis, approached the $1.3 billion annual sales mark in 2000 and is breaking away from the competition . . . Fosamax accounts for nearly 30 percent of the worldwide market for the treatment of osteoporosis, far ahead of its closest competitor.'[10]

Concerns are regularly raised about physicians who have financial relationships with the pharmaceutical industry because such relationships may pose a conflict of interest. As an example, an article published in the *New England Journal of Medicine* in 1998 reported on an extensive search of articles on the controversial calcium channel blockers — drugs used to treat hypertension. They found that authors who had financial relationships with the drug manufacturers were significantly more likely to support the use of the drugs than neutral or critical authors.[11]

The International Committee for Osteoporosis clinical guidelines for osteoporosis state that on the basis of accumulated evidence, Fosamax appears to be the most effective anti-fracture agent. They caution that Fosamax is expensive, and currently available evidence suggests it is cost-effective only when there is high risk of fracture.

A recent study measuring the effect of a new type of bisphosphonate called Risedronate (brand name Actonel) on hip fracture in 5,445 elderly women showed that it brought small benefit only. After three years of use, elderly women less than 80 years old with osteoporosis had a 1.9 percent incidence of hip fracture compared with 3.2 percent of the placebo group.[12] This translates to a hip fracture saving of just over one percent, so that if 100 women took the drug for three years, it would save just over one hip fracture. There has been no observed benefit in women over the age of 80, the age when they are at much higher risk for a hip fracture.

We assume that our doctors are fully aware of the benefits and risks that are associated with any drug they prescribe us. But in reality, most information on medications that doctors receive comes directly from the manufacturers, and although government regulations require that it is balanced and accurate, it sometimes falls short. A 1995 study published in the *Journal of the American Medical Association* which analysed more than

100 drug company rep statements found that 13 percent of their statements were inaccurate. The drug representative almost always made their drugs sound better than they were, and downplayed the side-effects.[13]

In *Perfect Blood Pressure Naturally* (Penguin, 2001) Dr David Lovell-Smith describes the carefully rehearsed strategies used by drug representatives when they visit doctors. Usually attractive, young, well presented and university-educated, they come offering gifts, empathy and information. But he warns that there is nothing innocently educational about the friendly overtures and the professional rapport. As well as promoting their product, they are there to gather detail '. . . about the doctor's family, prescribing habits, and reactions . . . later meticulously entered into a database that could be accessed by other members of [the] firm.' He goes on to say: 'Pharmaceutical company representatives are professional promoters. They are salespeople. It could be said that they cannot be blamed for using skills common to the world of selling. What is alarming however is that powerful sales techniques are being used to promote medicines that have considerable potential for harm . . . It is also of concern that the majority of medical people are untrained to recognise promotional techniques, nor do they realise how powerful and effective they are. The line between promotion and manipulation can easily become blurred.'[14]

Selective estrogen receptor modulators (SERMs)

The latest anti-osteoporosis treatment is Raloxifene, a drug known as a SERM or selective estrogen receptor modulator. As often happens with medicine, a drug prescribed for a certain purpose will show risks and benefits in unexpected ways. In the late 1980s, researchers noted that women taking Tamoxifen, a drug prescribed for those who have had breast cancer to prevent a recurrence, had increased bone density.

Since then a specific SERM called Raloxifene (Evista) has been developed that is anti-estrogenic — that is, it works in the opposite way to oestrogen in that it doesn't cause an increase of cancer cells in the classic target organs (for example, breast, uterus) but it has an anti-resorptive effect on bone, just as oestrogen does. Raloxifene is approved for prevention of postmenopausal bone loss. It is somewhat less effective as an antiresorptive drug than are oestrogens or bisphosphonates but studies have shown that it can prevent bone loss and possibly decrease the incidence of vertebral fractures. It is believed that it has the potential to produce some of the beneficial effects of oestrogen without the possible adverse effects. There is still much to be learned about SERMs and their mechanism of action, but predictions have been made that SERMs' share of the HRT market will climb from 3 percent in 1998 to 26 percent in 2008.[15]

At this stage there is limited evidence that Raloxifene reduces fracture rate. It has been found to prevent bone loss in recently menopausal women, and is believed to show great promise as a treatment option. But it can increase menopausal symptoms of hot flushing and leg cramps by 50 percent, and also poses an increased risk for venous thrombosis or clotting.

Interim data from the ongoing Multiple Outcomes of Raloxifene Evaluation (MORE) study involving 7,705 women, the largest osteoporosis trial ever performed, indicates that the selective oestrogen receptor modulator (SERM) reduced by about half the risk of new spinal fractures among post-menopausal women with low bone density, previous fractures or both, after 24 months of treatment.[16] Raloxifene also increased bone mineral density (BMD) by 2 percent to 2.5 percent, and decreased bone turnover over calcium and vitamin D alone (the control group). No change in the risk of non-vertebral fractures was observed. This study was funded by the drug company Eli Lilly which produces Evista, and the principal author disclosed a financial association with the company.

A recent television advertisement in the US drew criticism from the Food and Drug Administration (FDA) for Eli Lilly's claims of the benefits of the drug. The FDA charged the company with overstating the benefits and 'mis-characterising the nature of osteoporosis' by implying that the condition is itself debilitating and that all osteoporosis patients will suffer a fracture. The agency argued that the typical TV viewer would not understand from the advertisement that while osteoporosis increases the risk of fracture, not all patients will sustain fractures and even those who do will not necessarily have fractures with symptoms resulting in the 'loss of independence'. The FDA said that the TV spot implied 'outcomes and guarantees of efficacy' for Evista that were unsupported by clinical evidence, and inadequately disclosed the risks associated with its use.[17]

A 1999 advertisement in Canadian medical and pharmacy journals for Evista (Raloxifene) used the headline: 'A woman's choice for protecting her health' — a vague claim implying that all postmenopausal women could improve their health by taking the drug. The advertisement did not mention the risk of deep vein thrombosis or pulmonary embolism, although pre-marketing trials had associated these potentially fatal blood clotting disorders with the drug. There is also evidence of carcinogenity in animal trials, but there is no mention of this in the advertising fine print or on the labelling.[18] This advertisement went to doctors.

Calcitonin

Calcitonin is a hormone found naturally in our bodies. It is made by the thyroid gland and controls the activity of osteoclasts. Calcitonin has been used for many years in the prevention and treatment of osteoporosis — particularly in parts of Europe. This natural hormone has a good safety profile.

Calcitonin is considered a safe alternative for women who cannot or will not take oestrogen. The evidence supporting its anti-fracture use however is considered to be limited. Calcitonin has been used for the prevention of fractures and several studies provide evidence that it is a weak anti-resorptive agent with some anti-fracture efficacy. It also has a role in the management of severe pain due to vertebral crush fractures, apparently as a result of pain relief analgesic qualities which are separate from its effects on bone.[19]

Calcitonin is also found in certain fish, including salmon, and has been extracted for use as a drug to treat a bone disease called Paget's Disease, and in some cases, osteoporosis. A form of synthetic calcitonin in a nasal spray has been approved in more recent years for the treatment of osteoporosis in women who are five years postmenopause.

Nasal calcitonin is generally safe; the major adverse effect is local irritation. The most common side-effects are nasal symptoms (runny nose, crusting, nosebleeds), back and joint pain, and headache. Because calcitonin-salmon is a protein, the potential for a systemic allergic reaction exists. It is advised that the drug should be administered with adequate calcium and vitamin D (at least 400 IU daily).

When osteoporosis has occurred as a result of treatment from corticosteroids, calcitonin may be an effective treatment. A recent study showed that calcitonin appears to preserve bone mass in the first year of gluco-corticoid therapy at the lumbar spine by about 3 percent compared to a placebo, but not at the femoral neck (hip).[20]

Other treatments

Fluoride

There is considerable controversy about the effects of fluoride on bone strength and fracture risk. It is the only treatment known to stimulate osteoblast activity and actually increase bone mass as a result.

Dr Susan Ott says this about fluoride:

> In a large well-designed randomised, blinded clinical trial, women who used fluoride for four years had increased fracture rates compared to placebo controls. The bone density of the spine increased by 32 percent, but the hip did not show increased density and the rate of hip fractures was nearly three times as high in the fluoride group. At this time fluoride cannot be recommended for clinical use. Because it is one of the few medications that can enhance osteoblast activity, it thus deserves further research.[21]

There is some evidence that fluoridated water is linked to an increased risk of hip fracture, suggesting that low levels of fluoride may put elderly people at greater risk.[22] A 1995 study of elderly women in 75 parishes in south-western France found that the risk of hip fracture was 86 percent greater in those areas with water fluoride concentrations above 0.11 ppm.[23] This effect could be linked to the higher rate of fracture noted in clinical trials with fluoride.

Parathyroid hormone (PTH)

The role of parathyroid hormone in the control of bone mass is gaining new attention, and may be a treatment option for some people in the future. Being a hormonal treatment it is not without risks, however. Animal studies have shown long-term use is associated with bone cancer.

PTH stimulates osteoblast activity and bone formation, especially on trabecular bone surfaces. Patients with osteoporosis treated with PTH show increases at the spine but decreases at cortical sites. Recent studies using a combination of PTH and oestrogen in postmenopausal women have shown increased bone density at both the spine and the hip.[24]

Results have just been published of a very recent study of a PTH-based drug called Forteo produced by Eli Lilly. The study involved 1,637 postmenopausal women who had suffered at least one fracture. It is reported that the drug significantly reduced the risk of new fractures and significantly increased bone density. The drug is administered by injection.[25]

The study was stopped early because of a cancer scare resulting from other Eli Lilly research in which scientists found that rats developed bone cancer when given high lifelong doses of the drug. However, researchers eventually decided that the results did not suggest a higher cancer risk in people.

Growth hormone

Controversial human growth hormone treatment may soon be added to the list of treatment options for osteoporosis. A recent review of the evidence concludes that the increase of bone remodelling achieved with growth hormone may be helpful during late postmenopause when there is decreased bone turnover. Currently, however, results from studies are mixed, and its role in maintaining normal levels of bone density is uncertain. In some cases bone density has been shown to increase modestly. Using growth hormone to prevent physiological bone loss that occurs with age seems possible, but has to be debated more fully in terms of ethical and economic issues.[26]

Testosterone

Currently there is no evidence that hormone replacement or other hormone treatments like Raloxifene are beneficial for men. Testosterone treatment is increasingly being prescribed for men, although no studies of fracture efficacy have been done. Testosterone replacement is contraindicated in men who already have prostate cancer.

Calcitriol

Calcitriol is a derivative of vitamin D — necessary and important for the proper absorption and use of calcium in the body. Cacitriol is used along with oral calcium to prevent bone loss. There is preliminary evidence that calcitriol treatment may reduce vertebral fractures.[27]

As a metabolite of vitamin D, calcitriol increases the intestinal absorption of calcium, and has been advocated for the treatment of osteoporosis as it has been considered to stimulate bone formation.

There are dangers associated with use, mainly high levels of calcium in the urine and the potential for kidney damage with long-term use.

Progesterone

In recent years natural progesterone has become popular among many women and practitioners of natural medicine for the prevention and treatment of menopause symptoms and for the prevention of osteoporosis. Natural progesterone is synthesised in a laboratory from the wild yam or from soy. It is what is known as a 'nature identical' hormone because its molecular structure is identical to the hormone progesterone produced by the ovaries. In this way it differs from the synthetic progestogens (or progestins) used in HRT and hormonal contraceptives which have a slightly altered molecular structure.

There has been some evidence that progesterone enhances the formation of new bone.[28] Progestins (progestogens) used in HRT and contraceptives have been reported to prevent or reverse bone loss in certain clinical situations.[29] But in young women taking injectable medroxyprogesterone acetate (Depo-provera) for contraception, bone density was found to be 7 percent lower than young women not using the drug.[30]

The popularity of progesterone is based largely on the work and the writings of Dr John Lee, who reported that applying progesterone to the skin in the form of a cream was almost always successful in increasing bone mineral density in postmenopausal women.[31] Over a three-year period 100 women used the cream. Sixty-three of the women had bone density tests which indicated an average bone density increase of 15.4 percent over the period compared with an expected loss of 4.5 percent. Most of the women had previously fractured but no new fractures were reported over the period of the study. This was what is called an observational study — that is, there was no control group, so it does not rate as good evidence.

In addition to the progesterone, the women in the study were encouraged to consume leafy green vegetables, to avoid cigarettes and carbonated beverages, to supplement with calcium, vitamin D and vitamin C, and to participate in a regular exercise programme. Some of the women were also taking oestrogen. Because each of these additional recommendations may have a positive influence on bone density, it is difficult to say whether it was the progesterone or the combination of the strategies that had the effect.

In a more recent randomised controlled trial from the US involving 102 healthy postmenopausal women over one year, who used the progesterone cream and took calcium and vitamin supplements as well, there was no significant difference in bone density between the progesterone group and the control group.[32] The study did find that there was an 83 percent reduction in hot flushes in the women receiving progesterone compared with 19 percent in the placebo group — a benefit reported by many women who use the cream during the menopause transition.

Dr Alan Gaby, the author of the book *Preventing and Reversing Osteoporosis*,[33] has this to say of the outcome of the study:

> I believe it is still premature to conclude that progesterone has no role in osteoporosis prevention. The possibility remains that progesterone is biologically active only when administered as part of a comprehensive programme as recommended by Lee. Some practitioners of natural medicine have observed that administering the combination of transdermal progesterone and a 'bone building' nutritional supplement (that contains among other things, magnesium, vitamin K, vitamin C and trace minerals) will often increase bone mineral density in postmenopausal women, and that the effect of this combination is more pronounced than that of either treatment alone.

Longer-term studies involving such a multifactorial programme may therefore be warranted. In the meantime, however, it appears that transdermal progesterone either by itself or in combination with calcium and a multivitamin has little or no effect on bone mineral density.

DHEA

DHEA and DHEAS are steroid hormones secreted by the adrenal cortex and levels peak between the ages of 20 to 30 years. Levels decline steadily thereafter and at 70 years are found to be less than 20 percent of the peak when younger. Several studies have shown that supplementation with DHEA strengthens the immune system, heightens brain activity, and improves overall well-being. An increase in levels of oestrogen in postmenopausal women after supplementation with DHEA has been noted as a possible link to increasing bone density. At this time there are no studies to confirm the effect. As always, in the absence of long-term studies, concerns are raised about the safety of taking supplemental doses of the hormone.[34]

Ipriflavone

Many women are already using isoflavones made from soy and other plant sources for menopause, and as a protection against bone loss. Ipriflavone is a synthetic 'isoflavone' that until recently showed promise as an osteoporosis treatment.

Ipriflavone has been used in Japan since 1988. Soon afterwards it was registered in several other countries and has been used widely in Italy and Hungary. By 1997, 60 small studies involving 2,700 people had examined the effectiveness of ipriflavone. The combined evidence provided mainly positive evidence that ipriflavone prevented bone loss, and that it helped eliminate bone pain. It is a synthetic phytoestrogen, and thus acts in a similar way to phytoestrogens which are transformed into weak oestrogenic compounds in the body. Like phytoestrogens, ipriflavone does not appear to have any classical 'oestrogenic' effects such as stimulating breast or uterine tissue.

Data on the effectiveness of ipriflavone was conflicting, but generally showed that it would slow bone loss or increase bone mass in postmenopausal women. There was no conclusive evidence that it would prevent fracture. A recent large randomised controlled trial of 474 postmenopausal women — considered the definitive trial on ipriflavone — designed to investigate its effectiveness and safety found little to recommend it.[35] The women all had low bone density, and received either 600 milligrams (mg) of ipriflavone daily or a placebo daily for three years. In addition, all women took 500 mg of calcium daily.

No difference in bone density was seen between the two groups. However, in an adverse outcome, some of the women taking the ipriflavone had lower levels of certain white blood cells (lymphocytes) than those taking the placebo. Although this was a cause for concern, the study's lead author Peter Alexandersen reported that the women taking the ipriflavone did not show signs of lowered immunity by having more frequent attacks of cold or flu than women who took the placebo.

He concluded that although some small studies have suggested ipriflavone is effective in preserving bone mass, the current study found that 'in women at risk for osteoporosis, ipriflavone at these doses had no effect on bone density'.

Some health practitioners would recommend women eat more soy (of the non genetically-modified organic variety), which is rich in the isoflavonoids genistein and daidzein, as an alternative to ipriflavone.

CHAPTER NINE

The calcium dairy myth

DESPITE THE KNOWLEDGE THAT CALCIUM SUPPLEMEN-tation alone is not proven to build bone and that the countries with the highest rates of osteoporosis are the biggest consumers of dairy foods, both are named as essential weapons in the fight against the disease. The calcium and dairy industries have forged a place in the giant osteoporosis industry by bombarding women with the message that calcium supplements and a daily consumption of calcium-rich foods — preferably dairy products — are fundamental to the fight against osteoporosis.

Most people believe that diet has little to do with osteoporosis unless it relates to food that is high in calcium. It is extraordinary that the diverse nutritional needs of bone are ignored and that those at risk for osteoporosis are regularly advised to supplement with calcium alone. It is true that getting the recommended daily calcium intake at all ages is important, and preferably from dietary sources. But in fact most women with osteoporosis are getting plenty of calcium. Indeed, too much calcium can be harmful. Taken to excess it can cause kidney stones and gallstones. Many nutrients and mechanisms are involved in the building of peak bone mass in a young person, and even when there is a low calcium intake, a normal peak bone mass can be achieved.

Calcium has received the greatest attention because of its significant mass in the skeleton, and the rationale is that consuming a lot of calcium will make the bones stronger. But it is not that simple. Bones are complex, dynamic and alive, and have a wide range of nutritional needs. The ability to effectively absorb calcium can vary hugely, and excess calcium will be excreted from the body as a result of many factors.

A mature male skeleton contains more than 1,400 grams of calcium, and the female 1,200 grams. Ninety-nine percent of the total body calcium is found in the bones and teeth. The one percent circulating in the blood has significant functions, however. Calcium helps regulate heartbeat, nervous system function, muscle control, enzyme systems, and hormone secretions, and helps cells to cohere and blood to coagulate. If the body does not have enough circulating calcium for these functions, it takes it from the bones.

To sustain life, the level of calcium in the blood must be kept within a very narrow range. This is achieved by an exquisitely orchestrated mechanism involving parathyroid hormone and vitamin D, which maintains skeletal calcium and blood calcium in a state of equilibrium. Balance is maintained after adjusting for diet, intestinal absorption, excretion and hormonal functions as well as growth, physical activity and disease. For example, it is accepted that we always excrete about 150–250 mg of calcium per day, but it is also clear that this is affected by how much protein and sodium is consumed.

Because the amount of calcium in the bones is so carefully regulated by these hormones, increasing calcium intake is not going to fool them into building more bone. When researchers in Madison, Wisconsin, measured the diets and the bone density of 300 premenopausal women aged 20–39, they found that high calcium diets did not result in higher bone density.[1] In fact, too much calcium can be detrimental. Studies of countries with highest rates of hip fracture reveal that they also have the highest dietary intake of calcium — mainly from dairy products.[2]

It is well known that body calcium is controlled by calcitriol (vitamin D). Low levels of calcium will trigger an increase in levels of circulating calcitriol and improve calcium absorption, whereas high intakes will depress the levels of calcitriol and the calcium will be inefficiently used. People with high calcium diets have adapted and excrete more calcium than those with low intakes. With the wide variations in calcium intakes worldwide, this explains why osteoporosis is not rampant in those countries with low dietary calcium.[3]

Studies of children with low calcium and vitamin D intake in both developed and developing countries show that they still achieve a normal peak bone mass despite an apparently deficient diet. The author of a review of the evidence for this phenomenon comments, 'It is nearly impossible to explain the robust skeletal mass obtained by so many youngsters who have known nutritional inadequacies of calcium and vitamin D but who are otherwise healthy and active. Nature must somehow be providing well for skeletal growth despite limited intake of the critical nutrient calcium during periods of bone development.' He concludes: '. . . the beneficial effect of physical activity may dominate as a determinant of bone mass and bone density early in life.'[4]

Calcium absorption varies enormously from person to person. Clinical trials of postmenopausal women have found that calcium absorption can vary by as much as 61 percent, and that 40 percent of women in calcium balance trials could not absorb enough calcium to stay in balance even with an intake of 800 mg daily.[5] This could be due to high dietary salt or protein, for example, and highlights the importance of considering the multitude of other factors when treating osteoporosis. Poor intestinal absorption of calcium also occurs with celiac disease, or gluten intolerance, which remains undetected in many people.

If there is even a slight drop in blood calcium levels, this stimulates the release of calcium from the bones and its absorption from the intestine, at the same time decreasing its loss into the urine. The process is reversed through the actions of vitamin D, calcitonin, oestrogen, and other hormones. In this way bone mineral content is continuously being replenished.

The large body of clinical trials shows no relationship between supplemental calcium intake and bone density. Most studies have shown that calcium intake has little effect on the bone density of the spine, and none on the hip, the two places where most serious breaks can occur.[6] Seriously low calcium intake could lead to deficient bone formation, but calcium intake within the normal dietary range appears to be adequate. High dietary calcium intake has not been shown to lead to stronger bones.[7] The calcium intake in the Netherlands, for example, is high, and so is the incidence of osteoporosis.[8] In fact, low BMD, and a low dietary calcium intake, have been linked to fewer fractures in some countries. Especially in Asia and Africa (but also in the US and Europe) there are many people with low calcium intake, low BMD and healthy bones.

Better to limit calcium loss?

Taking calcium, whether as a supplement or via dairy products, seems to have little effect unless your diet is grossly calcium deficient. For the vast majority of people it seems that the answer lies in limiting calcium loss.

Food habits influence calcium requirements. Ingredients in food like phytates, oxalates and fibre can affect calcium absorption. Most importantly, the amount of protein and sodium (salt) we eat will affect how much calcium is lost in the urine. Protein from meat, milk, and eggs contains relatively high concentrations of sulphur amino acids which can increase calcium loss in the urine as urine becomes more acidic. Therefore, people who have low-protein or low-sodium diets may require lower calcium intakes than those on high-protein diets. A 1994 report in the *American Journal of Clinical Nutrition* showed that when animal proteins were eliminated from the diet, calcium losses were cut in half.[9]

The role of phosphorus in osteoporosis is unclear but it is believed that a dietary ratio of roughly an equal amount of calcium to phosphorus is necessary to maintain normal calcium levels. Because meat contains large amounts of phosphorus, excessive consumption of meat may therefore affect calcium balance. Phosphates in carbonated drinks can have a similar effect, and there is evidence that teenagers and children who consume carbonated drinks which are high in phosphoric acid have restricted calcium absorption. Researchers at the Harvard Medical School have found that cola drinks increase the fracture rates in young girls in the US.[10]

Smoking also causes calcium to be lost from the bone, and could result in a higher rate of fracture. In a study of the bone densities of identical twins, it was determined that long-term smokers had a 44 percent greater risk of fracture than their nonsmoking twins.[11]

It has also been found that people who reduce their salt (sodium) intake to 1–2 grams per day cut their calcium requirement by an average of 169 mg per day. For every gram of dietary salt consumed, approximately 26 mg of calcium is lost in the urine. And for each gram of animal protein consumed, one milligram of calcium is lost. That means that a 40 gram reduction in animal protein reduces the urinary loss by 40 mg which in turn, assuming about 20 percent is absorbed, lowers the requirement by 200 mg. This and the fact that people in developing countries tend to have more sunlight exposure and therefore get more vitamin D, can help explain the difference in fracture rates between cultures and between individuals. Some experts believe there is no single, universal calcium requirement, but one that is linked to a person's intake of other nutrients, in particular animal proteins and sodium.[12]

And a recent study of women in Pittsburgh, Pennsylvania, confirmed that taking a calcium supplement is only part of the story — having the body absorb it is another. Researchers found that the intake of fat and fibre significantly influences calcium absorption. Surprisingly, the women with a higher fat intake and a lower intake of fibre absorbed more calcium. Only certain types of fibre like wheat bran seem to reduce calcium absorption though — other forms such as the fibre found in green leafy vegetables such as kale, broccoli and bok choy did not appear to be detrimental. Women with high blood levels of vitamin D also showed increased absorption, while women with high alcohol intake showed decreased absorption.[13]

Calcium intake alone does not protect against osteoporosis. Nor does low calcium intake predict fracture risk. A 1992 review of fracture rates in many different countries showed that populations with the lowest calcium intakes had far fewer fractures than those with higher intakes.[14] For example, black South Africans had a very low average calcium intake — only 196 milligrams — yet their fracture incidence was far below that of either black or white Americans.

Consider these facts:

- Osteoporosis incidence (low bone density) is highest in those countries where the most (dairy) calcium is consumed: the USA, Australia, New Zealand, Switzerland, the UK and Northern Europe.[15]

- A study of Chinese women with osteoporosis found that, compared to the healthy control group, osteoporotic women appeared to have both a higher dietary calcium absorption rate and a higher calcium excretion rate.[16]

- In Gambia, bone mineral density, calcium intake and osteoporosis (fracture) incidence are very low.[17]

- African Bantu women take in only 350 mg of calcium per day, compared to the recommended daily amount of 1,200 mg. They bear an average of nine children during their lifetime and breast-feed them each for an average of two years. They never have calcium deficiency, seldom break a bone, and rarely lose a tooth. They consume much less calcium and much less protein than western populations, and yet are essentially free of osteoporosis (fractures).[18] And it can't be attributed to genes. Genetic relatives of the Bantus living in the US and eating the standard American diet have levels of osteoporosis-related fracture equal to those of their white neighbours.[19]

- Inuit peoples have a normal to very high dietary calcium intake (from 500 to 2,500 mg a day) and one of the world's highest protein intakes (from 250 to 400 grams a day) in the form of caribou, sea mammals, fish and birds. They also have one of the very highest rates of osteoporosis in the world.[20]

Dairy and bone

A lifetime of indoctrination from powerful media and advertising endorsement has made milk consumption to prevent fracture an institution in western countries. Yet these are the countries with the highest rates of osteoporosis (low BMD) and fracture.

Dairy foods have not been part of the diet of humans for most of human evolution. The Stone Age hunter-gatherers had a high calcium diet — derived largely from wild plants with high calcium content. It was not until the advent of the Agricultural Age some 10,000 years ago that animals became domesticated and in some parts of the world dairy products began to be introduced to babies after weaning.

For decades the dairy industry has convincingly marketed milk as the osteoporosis solution, and the public has trustingly believed them. Most baby-boom New Zealanders remember the daily trial as a child of having to swallow the half pint of warm milk provided free in schools, believed to offer the ultimate in nutritional requirements to the growing body. Yet this same generation is now being targeted as the osteoporosis 'at risk' population. Meanwhile, the dairy industry, blind to the irony, carries on publicising the supposed benefits of milk to bone. The dairy industry is burgeoning in New Zealand, and what better cause to push than bone strength to a society convinced that it is at risk for osteoporosis? Especially when fears of high cholesterol and high-fat diets have driven many away from dairy products like butter and cheeses.

Misleading advertising?
These days there is a huge marketing campaign underway to promote the milk and bone strength connection. The trolleys in our local supermarket currently have an advertisement cleverly placed inside to encourage you to pick up a few cartons of calcium-fortified milk on your way.

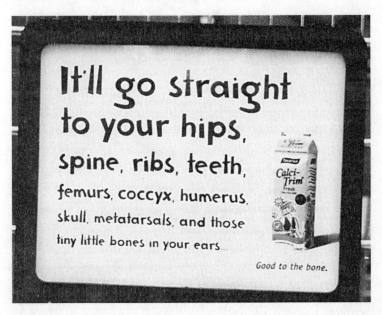

It'll go straight to your hips, spine, ribs, teeth, femurs, coccyx, humerus, skull, metatarsals, and those tiny little bones in your ears...

Calci-Trim

Good to the bone.

And on the way home from the supermarket there is a large billboard image of a carton of calcium-fortified milk. Last week it said, 'Best before: kick-boxing.' The week before it was, 'Best before: you slip in the bath.'

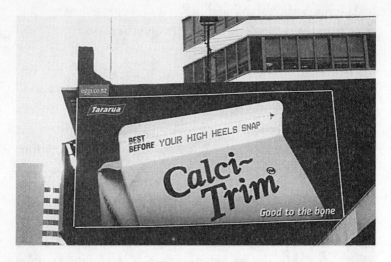

Even though it is well known that the countries consuming the most dairy products have the highest rates of fracture, the connection fails to be made, and the dairy industry has as big a foothold in the osteoporosis industry as the HRT industry does. Dairy products are said to provide about 70 percent of the dietary calcium of the US population.[21]

The dairy industry in the US spends hundreds of millions of dollars each year on advertising — using movie stars and celebrities as influential as President Clinton in their 'milk moustache' advertisements on television. It can come as a shock therefore to learn that dairy products could actually contribute to bone loss and fracture. Numerous studies published in prestigious journals like the *American Journal of Public Health* suggest that milk is ineffective in preventing osteoporosis.

Probably the most highly regarded of these is part of the famous Nurses' Health Study. It is difficult to argue with a trial so large and so well constructed, yet most people have no idea that it exists or that it provides the strongest evidence yet against the use of milk for bone health.

The study compared milk and calcium consumption in 77,000 women over a 12-year period in relation to the incidence of hip and forearm fractures. It found that those with the highest consumption of dairy products *had more fractures* than those who drank less milk. The authors concluded: 'These data do not support the hypothesis that higher consumption of milk and other food sources of calcium by adult women protects against hip or forearm fractures.'[22] A study of elderly residents in Australia reached the same conclusion. By reviewing their life-time dietary history, it found that consumption of milk and cheese in a person of age 20 years may increase the rate of hip fracture when that person becomes at risk in old age.[23]

A very recent review of 57 studies examining the evidence for dairy foods and bone health found that the majority of outcomes showed no significant relationship between the two. The authors conclude: '. . . the body of scientific evidence appears inadequate to support a recommendation for daily intake of dairy foods to promote bone health in the general US population.'[24]

Many studies are funded by the dairy industry, which has the money to support large numbers of researchers and can therefore determine what is studied and how it is presented. Given the funding source of these studies, it is hardly surprising that they come out in favour of drinking milk. When the results are reported in the popular press, the association with dairy industry funding is rarely made.

The focus on Asia

Meanwhile, ignoring conclusive evidence to the contrary, the US, European, Australian and New Zealand dairy industries have set about convincing the Asian market that dairy consumption will help reverse the pending 'epidemic' of osteoporosis there. Asian populations traditionally have very low consumption of dairy foods, and much less incidence of fragility fracture. This has been linked to traditional diets high in soy isoflavones and bone-building nutrients like vitamin K. Changing a traditional diet which has proven to be beneficial by introducing dairy foods raises many questions as to safety and usefulness given the lack of evidence that it will help to prevent fracture.

The New Zealand Dairy Board, which currently has a monopoly on exports to Asia, is establishing a massive market on the strength of two small trials which are said to prove that milk consumption increases bone density and reduces hip fracture amongst Asian women.

The trials were funded by the Dairy Board and conducted in Hong Kong by Professor Edith Lau from the Chinese University of Hong Kong. The first trial involved 200 Chinese women, half of whose diet was supplemented with two 200 ml glasses of a high-calcium milk powder drink per day over a 24-month period, and the other half who did not drink the product. The study is reported to show that drinking two glasses of the milk drink per day reduced the mean rate of bone loss at the lumbar spine by 72 percent and over the total body by almost 90 percent. Details of the second trial are unavailable. Although the two studies are referred to in a press release to the NZ media in 2000, at the time of writing, both remain unpublished.[25]

Claiming a world first in osteoporosis prevention following the trials, the New Zealand Dairy Board has launched a campaign to sell its products in Asia, Africa, the Middle East, the Indian sub-continent and South America. A 'clinically proven campaign' for the milk product was successfully launched in the Philippines and Malaysia through symposiums which were run for health professional audiences. Marketing also included TV commercials, special packaging, and supermarket promotions which have directly targeted consumers. Mostly unused to eating dairy foods, Asian children are being enticed by squeezable tubes of yoghurt, and something called Cheez Toys — cheese wrapped like confectionery and sold at supermarket checkouts.

New Zealand's new Global Dairy Company stands to be the world's ninth-biggest dairy company. Total revenue from the exported New Zealand-developed milk powder alone was around a quarter of a billion NZ dollars in the year 2000.

Asia and osteoporosis

Rates of osteoporosis-related fracture are low in Asia, as are rates of breast and prostate cancer. In 1996 the incidence of hip fracture in mainland China was still one of the lowest in the world. As Hong Kong has undergone increasing urbanisation, hip fractures there have increased to the point of doubling in the last 50 years. The reasons given for this are low calcium, lack of exercise, cigarette smoking, alcoholism and the increasing use of oral and inhaled steroids.[26] Much of Asian urbanisation involves the adoption of western foods and lifestyle trends. Accordingly the 'western' diseases of breast and prostate cancer are on the rise in countries like Singapore and Hong Kong. Hong Kong now has three times the rate of breast cancer of mainland China.[27] A study of Japanese women who had emigrated to the US found that when western-style diet and lifestyle was adopted, the incidence of oestrogen-dependent cancers like breast cancer increased.[28]

Traditional Asian diets are rich in calcium. Asian people live mostly on vegetables, a little fruit, and soybeans. They are not exposed to refined white flour, white sugar, carbonated drinks, and excessive red meat that modern research demonstrates reduces bone density and is linked to fractures. In addition, a great many Asian women eat a vegetarian diet, which is the preferred diet to maintain healthy bone.

Dairy foods are disliked

Dairy foods are not traditional foods in Asia. Many people are lactose-intolerant in China, and do not even use cow's milk to feed their babies. Culturally, the Chinese people are not accustomed to eating milk products and are apparently bemused by our preoccupation with milk and milk products.

In her book, *Your Life in Your Hands*, Professor Jane Plant, scientist and breast cancer survivor, tells this story:

> I remember entertaining a large delegation of Chinese scientists shortly after the ending of the cultural revolution in the 1980s. On advice from the Foreign Office, we had asked the caterer to provide a pudding that contained a lot of ice cream. After enquiring what the pudding consisted of, all of the Chinese including their interpreter, politely but firmly refused to eat it and they could not be persuaded to change their minds.[29]

Friend Diane recently returned from three months of voluntary primary nursing in the villages of south-east Cambodia, near the border with Vietnam. She reports having seen no evidence of osteoporosis in the elderly population. She also confirms a total lack of dairy products in the diet of these rural people:

'Even the buffalo are not milked. The diet is quite simply rice, vegetables and meat. Other than the availability of yoghurt in some supermarkets in Phnom Penh, dairy food is not in evidence.'

There is milk, and there is milk

Milk may not be the healthy food we think it is. A few sobering facts:

- Dairy products, with the exception of skim products, are loaded with saturated fat that is directly related to heart disease. Dairy products are also very high in protein, which is linked to calcium loss.

- Insulin-dependent diabetes is linked to dairy products. Studies show a strong correlation between the consumption of dairy products and the incidence of insulin-dependent diabetes.[30]

- Many people are allergic to milk. More than 50 million Americans and over 70 percent of the world's adult population are unable to digest the milk sugar lactose, which means they are lactose intolerant.[31, 32]

- Because of the artificial, high-pressure environment they are forced to live in, and without their calves which are removed at birth, there is a high incidence of mastitis and other infections in milking cows. Jane Plant points out that 'even in the European Union, milk for human consumption can be sold legally even when it contains up to 400,000 somatic pus cells/ml. So one teaspoon of milk can contain 2 million pus cells.'[33]

- For this reason, cows are routinely fed antibiotics. These are then passed directly on to the milk drinkers. A 1990 US FDA survey found antibiotics and other drugs in 51 percent of milk samples taken in 14 cities.[34]

- For Americans there is an even greater concern. On 23 January 1998 researchers at the Harvard Medical School released a major study providing conclusive evidence that IGF-1 or insulin-like growth factor 1 is a potent risk factor for prostate cancer. The milk of cows injected with synthetic bovine growth hormone (rBGH) to increase milk production has high levels of IGF-1. In his 1996 article in the *International Journal of Health Sciences*, Dr Samuel Epstein of the University of Illinois warned of the danger of high levels of IGF-1 in milk. He postulated that IGF-1 in rBGH-milk could be a potential risk factor for breast and gastrointestinal cancers as well as prostate cancer.[35]

In 1985 the Food and Drug Administration (FDA) in the United States approved the sale of milk from cows treated with rBGH (also known as BST) in large-scale veterinary trials and in 1993 approved commercial sale of milk from rBGH-injected cows. At the same time the FDA prohibited the special labelling of the milk so as to make it impossible for the consumer to distinguish between rBGH and non-rBGH affected milk.

Many of the contaminants and risks may be avoided by drinking organic low-fat milk.

Calcium or not?

Calcium is an essential nutrient. While it is uncertain how much calcium is actually needed, it is certain that diet affects calcium balance. Calcium supplements are not the best way to control osteoporosis for most people. A diet that is modest in protein and complemented by exercise is much more effective. Green leafy vegetables and beans are good sources of calcium that are also moderate in protein and very low in fat. Dark green vegetables, such as broccoli and collard, mustard, and turnip greens are much better sources of calcium than milk. A single cup of broccoli contains almost a fourth of the US recommended daily amount of calcium. For more on calcium-rich foods and food sources of other essential bone nutrients see Chapter 10.

CHAPTER TEN

Dietary and nutritional factors

I F BONE IS CONSTANTLY BEING DISSOLVED AND REBUILT, and part of that process involves various nutrients and the laying down of minerals extracted from the blood supply, our everyday diet must have a significant effect on bone health. Yet achieving the optimum dietary intake of essential nutrients may not be as easy as eating what appears to be a 'balanced diet'. For example, many of the foods we eat are grown on mineral-deficient soil, so they are not as nutritious as they appear. And consuming too much meat protein and drinking too much coffee or coke could cause bone loss, not gain.

Most of the foods that are known to be beneficial offer many of the bone nutrients simultaneously. For example, many of the foods high in calcium are also high in phytoestrogens, vegetable protein, protective antioxidants, essential bone-building minerals, and vitamins. Increasing your intake of leafy greens, sea vegetables, non-starchy vegetables, nuts and seeds, and reducing your intake of meat protein, dairy, salty foods and carbohydrates, creates a bone-nutrient rich, alkaline-producing diet that reduces calcium excretion and thereby the need for supplements.

A recent investigation of the diets of elderly men and women in Framingham, Massachusetts, found that those people who had greater intakes of potassium, magnesium and of fruit and vegetables had less decline in bone mass in the hip and forearm than those elderly people who ate less of these foods.[1]

Phytoestrogens

Phytoestrogens are plant compounds that are structurally similar to the oestrogen which is produced by the human ovaries. Yet they don't work exactly like oestrogens. Their effect is more subtle and they appear to have an oestrogenic (proliferative) and non-oestrogenic action. Phytoestrogens are of increasing interest because they have a multitude of hormone-like properties that can be beneficial to women. There is growing evidence that regular consumption of fruits, vegetables, grains and legumes rich in plant hormones can positively influence a woman's health and hormone balance.

There is also evidence that a regular diet of phytoestrogen-rich foods may decrease menopause symptoms including hot flushes, help prevent osteoporosis, and help reduce the incidence of heart disease.[2, 3, 4] Although there is limited and uncertain evidence around their safety in regard to oestrogen-fed cancers like breast and prostate, it is noted that these diseases are low in communities with a soya-based diet.[5, 6]

Phytoestrogens are divided into several classes, but current research and interest focuses on isoflavones (found in soy and red clover) and lignans (found in oilseeds and cereals). Phytoestrogens are known to be transformed by bacteria present in the intestine into active compounds in the bloodstream that have a weak oestrogenic effect.[7] However, it is known that there is large variation among individuals in their bowel metabolism of phytoestrogens, which could be due to a lack of the necessary bacteria, or to antibiotic use. This means that some people may experience more benefit than others.

The traditional diets of approximately half the world's population contain moderate to high levels of phytoestrogens. In Asian cultures women traditionally have a diet which is low in fat, high in fibre and rich in a wide variety of fresh fruit and vegetables (phytoestrogens), in contrast to the high protein, carbohydrate and fat diet more typical of the western diet. A study of Japanese women who had emigrated to the US found that when western-style diet and lifestyle were adopted, the incidence of oestrogen-dependent cancers like breast cancer increased.[8]

A dietary survey of 1,106 Japanese women found that the consumption of soy products was also effective in preventing hot flushes.[9] The authors noted that although HRT is effective in treating hot flushes, Japanese women in general prefer not to take it and would rather manage menopause in a natural way.

There is increasing evidence that soy in particular has an effect on bone density, but there is still no evidence for fracture prevention. A recent Hong Kong study of 130 women aged 30–40 indicated that a high soy intake appears to reduce the rate of bone mineral density decline in premenopausal Chinese women. Women consuming the highest amount of soy had the lowest rate of bone loss. Principal researcher Dr Suzanne C. Ho, who was speaking at the Third Annual Scientific Meeting of the Hong Kong

Epidemiological Association in 2001, commented that 'soy intake does appear to be a factor involved in bone mineral density, along with genetic factors, and other dietary components such as calcium, protein, vitamin C and iron intake. We also believe that soy intake can influence the attainment of peak bone mass.' She added that many Chinese women are considering soy as an alternative to hormone replacement therapy.[10]

A similar recent study of 85 Japanese women also indicated that high soy protein intake is associated with a higher bone mineral density and a lower level of bone resorption. The authors noted that further studies are needed to confirm just how soy has this effect.[11]

A randomised controlled trial found that women taking 40 grams of soy protein powder per day (equivalent to 90 mg isoflavones per day) increased bone mineral density of the spine.[12] However, lower intakes (providing 56 mg isoflavones per day) did not improve bone density in this report. The study lasted only six months but results suggested that higher-dose soy isoflavones may prevent bone loss in postmenopausal women. Isoflavones from soy have been found to protect animals from bone loss.[13]

Soy foods such as tofu, tempeh, miso, soy milk, roasted soy beans and soy extract powders are rich sources of isoflavones.

Others are:

- legumes — chickpeas, lentils, beans (mung, haricot, broad, kidney and lima)

- wholegrain cereals — wheat, wheatgerm, barley, hops, rye, rice, bran, oats

- fruit — cherries, apples, pears, stone fruits, rhubarb

- seeds — linseed or flaxseed, sunflower, anise, sesame
- vegetables — green and yellow vegetables, carrots, fennel, onion, garlic
- ginseng, liquorice.

Soy is controversial

These days there are many concerns about what is perceived as the multi-million dollar misuse of soy. Soy is being genetically modified (GM) to be resistant to herbicides and now floods the global market in its altered form. The effect of this and the altered genetic material on humans who consume it is unknown and untested. To avoid consuming GM soy, it is necessary to eat food labelled organic, which at present does not contain genetically engineered products.

GM soy is used as a bulk additive in processed foods, and it is estimated that about 60 percent of foods including margarine, cakes, ice-cream, pasta, pizza bases, biscuits and mayonnaise have soy flour added. In the absence of labelling which identifies the presence of GM ingredients, it might be better to look to many other possibly safer plant sources for your daily intake of phytoestrogens.

There have been warnings in New Zealand against feeding soy milk to infants, as large quantities of even weak plant hormone may be inappropriate for children. The effect of suddenly adding large quantities of soy (particularly soy milk) to the adult diet is also unknown. It could be that as soy foods are relatively new to western digestive systems, we may not have evolved to cope with them as well as our Asian counterparts.

Traditional methods of preparation of soy, which involved a long process of fermentation, have been abandoned in favour of a quicker form of processing. Today's soy milk, for example, is produced by soaking the beans in an alkaline solution, then heating them up to about 115 degrees Celsius. This produces difficult-to-digest proteins, plus phytates that block the essential uptake of minerals. The traditional methods of preparation reduced soy's mineral-robbing 'anti-nutrients' and improved its digestibility. The only modern commercial soy foods that undergo this fermentation are good-quality tempeh (not tofu) and miso (not soy sauce).

Other dietary considerations

Protein

Cutting back on meat protein is essential. Animal protein tends to leach calcium from the bones, leading to its excretion in the urine. Animal proteins are high in sulphur-containing amino acids. Sulphur is converted to sulphate, which tends to acidify the blood. During the process of neutralising this acid, calcium from bone dissolves into the bloodstream and filters through the kidneys into the urine. Meat and eggs have two to five times more of these sulphur-containing amino acids than are found in plant foods.[14]

Protein from vegetables is preferable. A 1994 report in the *American Journal of Clinical Nutrition* showed that when animal proteins were eliminated from the diet, calcium losses were cut in half.[15] A very recent study of older white American women found that those who consumed a diet high in animal protein had a more rapid loss of bone from the hip, and a greater risk of hip fracture. The authors suggest that an increase in vegetable protein could reduce that risk.[16] Protein is important for bone health and approximately 20 grams a day is recommended. Vegetable protein is found in grains, nuts, beans, vegetables and fruit.

Another study followed over 85,000 American women for 12 years. Those who ate the most animal protein (meat and poultry and dairy) had a significantly higher risk of osteoporotic fractures.[17] When meat protein consumption is high then more calcium is required as well. Reducing meat and dairy intake and adopting a vegetarian diet with an adequate protein component is an option. Low protein intakes in developing countries may account for the lower rates of fracture in those countries.

Sodium (salt)

Although a definite link between salt intake and fracture risk has not yet been established, increases in dietary salt have shown an increase in the loss of calcium in the urine. People who reduce their sodium intake to 1–2 grams per day cut their calcium requirement by an average of 60 mg per day.[18] Most nutrition experts therefore recommend less salt and less highly salted foods.

Caffeine

There is conflicting evidence that caffeine intake is linked to osteoporosis. In one trial caffeine was linked with lower bone mass, but only in women who consumed relatively little calcium.[19] The authors of this report concluded that two to three cups of coffee per day might speed bone loss in women with calcium intakes of less than 800 mg per day. A more recent study of women aged 55–70 who had no risk factors for osteoporosis showed no link between caffeine intake and loss in bone density.[20] There is no evidence that coffee intake is linked to fragility fractures. Most nutritional experts recommend restricting your coffee consumption to one cup a day.

Vitamin D

Sunlight is the best source of vitamin D, although some countries produce fortified milk which can boost the body's supply. Other sources include herring, mackerel, salmon, sardines, and cod- and halibut-liver oils.

Women and men who don't get sun exposure and who eat less than four servings a day of fortified food should take a daily multivitamin which contains 400 units of vitamin D. But even that may not be enough for those who are house-bound elderly patients or confined to nursing homes. A recent study of elderly people found that the majority had low levels of the nutrient even though most of them were taking multivitamins containing 400–800 IU of vitamin D daily.[21]

After the age of 70 the skin does not convert vitamin D as effectively, so dietary sources become even more important. Many experts now feel that older men and women should be getting 1000 units/day of vitamin D. Doses of 50,000 IU per day can prove toxic.

Magnesium

Magnesium's role in bone health appears to be significant, so it is curious that it is routinely overlooked in the rush to recommend calcium supplementation. As much as 50 percent of all the magnesium in the body is found in the bones. Many researchers are now reporting that magnesium deficiency is very common and that it plays a big part in the development of osteoporosis (low bone density).

Studies have shown that women with low bone density tend to have a lower intake of magnesium than normal and also have lower levels of magnesium in their blood and in their bones.[22] A trial in Israel showed that postmenopausal women with osteoporosis (low BMD) could stop further bone loss by supplementing with 250–750 mg/day of magnesium for two years.[23] Some (8 percent) even experienced a significant increase in bone density. Untreated controls lost bone density. Another study in Czechoslovakia found that 65 percent of women who supplemented with 1500–3000 mg of magnesium lactate daily for two years were rid of their pain and stopped further development of deformities of the vertebrae.[24]

A recent Austrian study of magnesium supplementation in young males found indications that magnesium suppressed high bone turnover, which could be beneficial in reducing associated bone loss.[25]

An Australian study looking at the relation of a mother's diet during pregnancy to her children's BMD, found that spinal bone density was significantly higher with the highest maternal intake of phosphorus, magnesium and potassium. BMD was lower with a high maternal fat intake. According to the researchers, total body BMD was significantly associated with magnesium only.[26]

It could be that magnesium deficiency is a reflection of modern life. In his book *Preventing and Reversing Osteoporosis*, Alan Gaby addresses the function and role of magnesium. He comments, 'Physical, emotional and chemical stresses probably caused by the release of adrenaline, draw magnesium out of the cells allowing it to be flushed out in the urine.'[27]

Magnesium is important for calcium regulation. Although the optimum ratio of calcium to magnesium is not established, there is evidence that two parts calcium to one part magnesium will allow for better calcium absorption. Milk apparently has four parts calcium to one part magnesium.[28]

Magnesium influences bone metabolism and if levels become depleted, bone growth stops. A magnesium deficiency can also affect the production of the biologically active form of vitamin D and thereby further promote osteoporosis. In a review of the available literature on the role of magnesium, the authors comment, 'There is growing evidence that magnesium may be an important factor in the qualitative changes of the bone matrix that determine bone fragility.'[29] They note that bone mineral with decreased magnesium content results in larger, abnormally shaped bone crystals which may be more brittle than smaller, normal crystals, and add: 'Trabecular bone from osteoporotic women has a reduced magnesium content and larger bone crystal formation than controls.'

The US recommended daily amount of magnesium is 350 mg, but a typical American diet contains only about 250 mg. Some researchers believe that the optimal daily intake of this mineral is more than 600 mg. Magnesium is found in many foods (see table page 176).

Calcium sources

While the popular exclusive focus on calcium intake is inappropriate, the body does need calcium, and it is best to source it from food. The optimal calcium intake is not known. The World Health Organisation recommends 400–500 milligrams of calcium per day for adults. The American recommended daily amount is higher, at 800 milligrams per day or even more, partly because the meat, salt, tobacco, and physical inactivity of American life leads to rapid calcium loss.

The best absorbed calcium sources are green leafy vegetables and legumes. They have several advantages that dairy products lack. Dairy contains animal protein, and has comparatively low levels of magnesium. Vegetables and legumes contain antioxidants, complex carbohydrates, fibre, and iron, and have little fat and no cholesterol.

Calcium absorption from vegetables is better than that from milk. Calcium absorption from milk is approximately 32 percent, but is possibly offset by the negative effect of acid-forming protein. Calcium absorption from broccoli, Brussels sprouts, mustard greens, turnip greens and kale ranges from 40–64 percent.[30] Spinach is an exception. It contains a large amount of calcium, but in a form that is poorly absorbed due to the presence of oxalic acid. Beans (for example, pinto beans, black-eyed peas and navy beans) and bean products, such as tofu, are rich in calcium and vegetable protein. Seaweeds contain high amounts of calcium, phosphorus, magnesium, boron, iron, iodine and sodium. They also contain vitamins A, B1,C, E, and are one of the few vegetarian sources of B12.

Calcium and magnesium in foods (milligrams)

Source	Calcium	Magnesium
Barley (1 cup)	57	158
Bok choy (1 cup)	250	
Broccoli (1 cup, boiled)	180	38
Brown rice (1 cup, cooked)	20	86
Brussels sprouts (8 sprouts)	56	32
Butternut squash (1 cup, boiled)	84	60

Chickpeas (1 cup, cooked)	80	78
Dates (10 medium, dried)	27	29
Figs (10 medium, dried)	269	111
Green beans (1 cup, boiled)	58	32
Kale (1 cup, boiled)	200	24
Kidney beans (1 cup)	115	
Lentils (1 cup, boiled)	37	71
Lima beans (1 cup, boiled)	32	82
Mustard greens (1 cup, boiled)	150	20
Navel orange (1 medium)	56	15
Navy beans (1 cup, boiled)	128	107
Oatmeal (1 cup)	326	70
Pinto beans (1 cup, boiled)	82	95
Raisins ($\frac{2}{3}$ cup)	53	35
Soybeans (1 cup, boiled)	175	148
Tofu ($\frac{1}{2}$ cup)	258	118
Vegetarian baked beans (1 cup)	128	82
White beans (1 cup, boiled)	161	113

Vitamin K

Bone contains significant amounts of vitamin K, and low blood levels have been found in those with osteoporosis and in postmenopausal women. Vitamin K is required for the production of osteocalcin, the protein which attracts calcium to bone tissue and facilitates beneficial calcium crystal formation. Vitamin K supplements have been shown to increase this process (known as carboxylation) in postmenopausal women, thereby reducing bone loss. In controlled trials, people with low bone density given large amounts of vitamin K (45 mg per day) showed an increase in bone density after six months and decreased bone loss after one year.[31]

Insufficient vitamin K could be linked to fracture. Research at Harvard University found that women who consumed less than 109 mcg a day sustained 30 percent more hip fractures over a ten-year period.[32]

In the Framingham heart study between 1988 and 1995, 888 elderly men and women consumed various levels of vitamin K. Those averaging 56 mcg experienced more hip fractures by 1995 than those reporting the highest intake levels of 254 mcg. Researchers stated that vitamin K activates at least three proteins involved in bone health.[33]

It has long been known that astronauts lose bone density rapidly in space. Scientists recently identified that there is a lack of vitamin K in astronauts, which may directly cause the space-related bone loss.[34]

Because 90 percent of the vitamin K in the liver is made by intestinal bacteria, anyone who has had frequent or long-term antibiotic use is likely to have insufficient vitamin K. Vitamin K is fat soluble and can be malabsorbed by those with chronic malabsorption or gastrointestinal problems. Broccoli is a great source of vitamin K, as are other leafy greens, legumes, and soybean oil.

Manganese

Manganese is a trace mineral required for bone mineralisation and the formation of connective tissue in cartilage and bone. In a small study of Belgian women with osteoporosis (low BMD), blood levels of manganese were 75 percent lower than those of women without osteoporosis.[35] In a now famous case, US top basketball player Bill Walton's repeated fractures ceased when he supplemented with manganese.[36] Author Alan Gaby comments: 'Evidence suggests that the manganese content of our diet is lower than in previous generations; that adulteration of our food and pollution of our environment may be interfering with absorption or utilisation of manganese. Manganese . . . may be a significant factor contributing to the increasing incidence of osteoporosis.'[37] Manganese is toxic in high doses. Between 15 and 20 mg daily is the recommended amount. Excellent sources of manganese include pecans, peanuts, pineapple fruit and juice, oatmeal, beans (pinto, lima, navy), rice, spinach, sweet potato, and whole wheat bread.

Zinc

Zinc, along with vitamin A and C, is essential for the formation of collagen. It also enhances the biochemical action of vitamin D. Zinc levels have been found to be low in elderly people with osteoporosis. In one study, men consuming only 10 mg of zinc per day had almost twice the risk of osteoporotic fractures compared with those with significantly more zinc in their diets.[38] It has not yet been proven that zinc supplementation will prevent osteoporosis but many doctors recommend that their patients supplement with 10–30 mg daily. Zinc is found in wholegrain products, wheat bran and wheat germ, brewer's yeast and pumpkin seeds.

Copper

Copper is needed for normal bone synthesis; it is a factor in the strengthening of connective bone tissue. A placebo-controlled two-year study reported that 3 mg of copper daily prevented bone loss.[39] Although more research is required to confirm the role of copper in treating osteoporosis, many nutritionists recommend 2–3 mg per day, especially if the person is supplementing with zinc, as zinc will deplete copper levels.

Strontium

Strontium, the trace mineral (not to be confused with the radioactive substance of the same name), plays a crucial role in bone remodelling. It tends to migrate to sites in bone where active remodelling is taking place. Preliminary evidence suggests that women with fragility fractures may have reduced levels of strontium. Several small studies have observed decreased bone pain and an increase in bone formation in people taking quite high doses of strontium.[40] Most experts recommend about 1–3 mg per day.

Boron

Boron is a trace element which appears to have an important role in bone building and strength. It plays a part in parathyroid metabolism and influences the functions of calcium and magnesium, vitamin D and phosphorus. Supplementation has been shown to increase the level of oestrogen in some women. In a 1987 study, women taking 3 mg of supplemental boron for 7 weeks lost 44 percent less calcium and 33 percent less magnesium in their urine than those not taking boron.[41] Boron deficiency has also been linked to arthritis and there are indications that supplemental boron may provide relief. In areas where soil levels of boron are high it has been noted that arthritis incidence is lower.[42]

More studies are needed into the role of this trace mineral. Boron is extremely safe when taken at the recommended dosage of 3 to 9 mg. It is found in the greatest concentration in avocados, followed by legumes and nuts. Boron is in good supply in most soils and food.

Silicon

Silicon is another trace mineral, important for skin and hair, and in the formation of connective tissue, bone and cartilage. It combines with calcium and is highly concentrated at sites of growing bones. In preliminary research, supplementation with silicon increased bone mineral density in a group of eight women with low bone density.[43] Silica is found in hard unprocessed grains and vegetables, especially cabbage, parsnips, asparagus and radishes, and fruits such as olives. Horsetail and oatstraw tea are excellent sources of silica. It may be beneficial to drink a cup per day.

Betain

Individuals with osteoporosis often absorb calcium poorly. Low stomach acid (hypochlorhydria) is relatively common in women over the age of 50 and may reduce absorption of most forms of calcium. Betain increases the absorption of bone-building nutrients.

Folic acid, vitamin B6, vitamin B12

These three are known to reduce levels of the amino acid homocysteine in the body. Homocystinuria, a condition associated with high homocysteine levels, is known to cause osteoporosis. Although no research exists on the effects of supplementation, normal amounts found in high-potency B-complex supplements should be adequate.[44] Pyroxidine (vitamin B6) is required for collagen linking and the strength of connective bone tissue.

Vitamins A and C

Your body uses these to make collagen, which keeps bones flexible and strong. Animal studies have shown that osteoporosis can result from vitamin C deficiency.[45] The suggested daily supplemental dose is 500mg.

Although daily dietary intake is essential, too much vitamin A could be harmful. In a Swedish study where 247 women with hip fracture were compared with 873 matched controls, every 1mg/day increase in vitamin A (retinol) intake increased the risk of hip fracture by 68 percent. While it is essential for the formation of collagen, the authors caution that excessive dietary intake of vitamin A is associated with reduced bone mineral density and an increased risk for hip fracture.[46]

Vitamin E

It is known that free radical activity may increase bone resorption. A preliminary report on the effectiveness of vitamin E in preventing bone loss in animals suggests that supplementation may be a way to reverse free radical damage in bone.[47]

Essential fatty acids

Supplementing with fish oil may improve calcium metabolism in older women with osteoporosis. A preliminary study of women of average age 80 with osteoporosis (low BMD) who took four grams of fish oil (gamma-linoleic acid) every day for four months found that they had higher blood levels of calcium, improved calcium absorption and chemicals in their urine indicating bone formation. And combined with evening primrose oil which also provides gamma-linoleic acid, there was an increase in bone density of 3.1 percent over a three-year period.[48] This is a significant outcome in older women, and more research is needed in this important area.

Bone care nutrients

A well-balanced diet provides the best source of nutrients. If your diet is inadequate, or you wish to make sure you are getting the essentials, you can make up the balance with a mineral and vitamin supplement.

There are many supplements available for bone and it can be confusing choosing the right one. Here is a basic combination of which you ought to be able to find an approximation in a health food store:

- Calcium: 400–1200 mg of calcium citrate at bedtime. Citrate is the most absorbable form of calcium. Calcium hydroxy-apatite is another source, but vegetarians need to be aware that it is derived from beef or calf bone. In the days of animal-borne diseases it could involve risk. Bone meal and oyster shell could also contain high levels of lead.

- Vitamin B6: 5–50 mg

- Folic acid: 0.4–5 mg

- Boron: 2–3 mg

- Copper: 1–2 mg

- Vitamin C: 100–1,000 mg

- Vitamin E: 400IU. Caution: if you are taking anticoagulants, you should not take vitamin E supplements.

- Vitamin D: 400 IU

- Magnesium: 400–800 mg

- Manganese: 5 mg

- Vitamin K: 100 to 500 micrograms

- Zinc: 10–30 mg. Do not exceed 80 mg.

- Silicon: 1–2 mg

- Strontium: 0.5–3 mg.

Summary

Although the true cause of brittle, fragile bones remains unclear, it is evident that at least in part it is tied to dietary and lifestyle issues. Because incidence of fracture is seen to vary widely from one culture to another, it is worthwhile considering the dietary differences between countries with a higher incidence and those with a lower incidence. Favouring fresh vegetables, leafy greens and vegetable proteins, and avoiding refined foods, heavy meats, caffeine and carbonated drinks is a fundamental prevention and treatment strategy. Ensuring adequate intake of essential bone nutrients is another. Both these approaches will benefit overall health as well as bone health, and coupled with a regular exercise programme may offer the most effective means to prevent bone loss and fragility fracture at this time.

CHAPTER ELEVEN

Exercise

E XERCISE BENEFITS THE SKELETON AND IS THE SINGLE most effective strategy to prevent fragility fracture. No other agent, hormonal or mineral, can actually cause the skeleton to become heavier or sturdier in response to the demands made of it. Bone formation is stimulated by the mechanical forces that exercise generates, particularly higher-impact activities like jogging, running and jumping, which generate more effect on bones than lower-impact exercise like swimming or walking.

The force of muscles pulling against bones promotes new bone growth. The more you use your muscles, the more this stimulates bone remodelling and bone formation. This effect has been repeatedly observed in athletes. A recent study of volleyball players demonstrated that top male players show remarkably high bone density in the hip and spine regions, and high bone density in their arms and legs. Interestingly, the volleyball 'smashing' arm was up to 9 percent more dense than the less involved arm, believed to be a result of the body's adaptation to the greater demands made on that arm.[1]

A recent review of all the randomised controlled studies done on exercise and bone mass in pre and postmenopausal women concluded that the studies consistently showed that exercise prevented or reversed about one percent of bone loss per year at both the spine and the hip.[2] There is also evidence that those with lowest BMD tend to show greatest response to exercise, so this is a great incentive for anyone with a BMD diagnosis of osteoporosis.[3]

Age is no barrier. People 80 years and over can reduce their risk of osteoporosis while also improving muscle tone and balance.[4] Exercise programmes offered by trained health professionals which target strength and balance, or strength and endurance, have been found to reduce the frequency of falls in high-risk older people. These programmes are in addition to walking activities and involve the gentle and gradual use of weights, and exercises to increase balance. A New Zealand home exercise programme delivered by trained nurses to 450 women and men aged 79–94 resulted in a significant reduction in the incidence of falls. Another slightly smaller programme produced similarly good results.[5, 6, *]

Physical activity is considered one of the most important factors in acquiring peak bone mass while young, and it is believed that modern trends of watching television and sitting

---

* There are other excellent spin-offs from such a strategy. My father was part of this programme. He conscientiously followed the exercise routines daily for several months and was able to increase significantly the size of the weights and the duration of use. Although he is a very fit person, his excellent recovery from a major surgical procedure (abdominal aortic aneurysm repair) could in part be a result of the level of strength and fitness achieved at the time.

in front of computers may be having a negative effect. High-impact exercise has been found to have the most beneficial effect on bone mass in girls before puberty, rather than after.[7]

Regular exercise has numerous other benefits. It increases well-being and fitness. It also helps protect against conditions like heart disease, cancer, depression and Alzheimer's disease.[8] In addition, weight training which increases overall strength can give a sense of competency when the performance of daily tasks like lifting, carrying groceries or pushing the lawn mower becomes much easier. Although weight training is not aerobic, it will help increase the metabolism, which in turn can help shed excess weight.

T'ai chi

Visit Auckland's Cornwall Park in the early morning and you will see older, predominantly Asian men and women gracefully executing their t'ai chi routines. Evidently very supple and able to balance on one leg then the other with ease, they move quietly in flowing, dance-like actions. For the full sensory impact of mass practice of this form of Chinese exercise, go to the Lumphini Park in Bangkok any day at dawn. Literally thousands of predominantly elderly people sorted into brightly clad groups perform their version of t'ai chi — with music competing from portable sound systems. The effect is astonishing and awe-inspiring.

T'ai chi enhances balance and body awareness through slow, graceful and precise body movements. Legend has it that in the 12th century a group of Chinese monks decided to try a new form of meditation — one which would imitate the rhythms of the world and the life all around them. T'ai chi was the result.

The main principle of t'ai chi is that it uses subtle movements that cause energy to flow in the body. According to traditional Chinese medicine, it is an excellent way of accumulating energy (chi), storing it, and then circulating it through the body to balance it and prevent or heal disease. Studies show that t'ai chi can improve strength, flexibility and endurance in patients suffering from osteoarthritis, that it is an excellent weight-bearing exercise which can decrease joint swelling and tenderness, and that it can improve balance and reduce the incidence of falls in men and women over 70 years.[9]

It is one of the few exercises which teaches how to bear all the body weight on one leg at a time and which thus promotes increased bone formation in the weight-bearing pelvic bones and femur. A US study of the effect of regular t'ai chi exercises over a 15-week period included 200 participants aged 70 and older who were living in the community. The participants were divided into groups for t'ai chi, computerised balance training, and education. The most notable outcome was a 47.5 percent reduction in the rate of multiple falls for the t'ai chi group. Fear of falling was also reduced. The groups receiving computerised balance training and education did not have significantly lower rates of falling.[10]

Commentators at the time noted that the success of t'ai chi is a reminder that relatively 'low tech' approaches should not be overlooked in the search for ways to prevent disability and maintain physical performance later in life. And it needn't take a lot of time — a mere ten minutes of t'ai chi practice a day is reported to be beneficial for most people who choose this exercise as a part of their health regimen. Once you have received qualified instruction, you can practise it successfully at home . . . or in your local park!

Sedentary lives

Lack of exercise and immobility will reduce bone density and general strength and fitness. Bedridden patients lose muscle and bone and have increased levels of urinary calcium, indicating that calcium is being lost from the bone.

A recent survey of adult New Zealanders revealed some interesting lifestyle facts. We spend an average of 40 minutes a day on grooming, one and a half hours socialising, one and a half hours eating, two hours watching TV and eight minutes exercising.[11] Life in the 21st century works against us being physically active. It continues to get easier to avoid exercising. Daily activity is geared towards working our bodies less and less as technology replaces physical effort. Many of us sit for hours in front of computer terminals and now send much of our mail electronically — threatening to deny us even the walk to the letterbox! Power steering in the car leaves arm muscles unexercised . . . escalators and lifts waft us from floor to floor and when we shop, car parks adjoin malls and shopping centres.

The National Aeronautics and Space Administration physicians discovered that weightless astronauts lost bone in space at the dizzying rate of 1.5 percent a month. Dr Norman Thagard spent 115 days in space on the Russian space station Mir. He lost 11.7 percent of his bone material and 17.5 pounds of overall muscle and weight during his sojourn. Most of this loss came from the hip and lower spine. Dr Frank M. Sulzman, director of life science research at NASA, says a trip to Mars, which takes a year or two each way, may leave an astronaut permanently crippled upon return to Earth.[12]

No group is at higher risk for depression, disease and early death than people who are completely sedentary. Studies from the Russian space programme also showed that young cosmonauts subjected to the forced inactivity of space flight fell prey to depression. When they were put on a schedule of regular exercise, the depression was avoided.[13]

Exercise and the older person

Physiologists used to believe that exercise benefits us primarily at young ages when muscles are in their prime developmental stage. However, research with the elderly has conclusively demonstrated that a person can take up exercise at any age — even centenarians will receive the same increase in strength, stamina and muscle mass as a younger person. Weight training in particular has special benefits for the frail elderly. In a 1992 study of frail, very elderly volunteers who were prone to falling easily, Maria Fiatarone and colleagues at the Hebrew Rehabilitation Center for Aged observed that, after adopting a regular resistance training programme, men and women tripled their thigh muscle mass and dramatically lowered their risk of falls.[14]

In 1990 researchers from Tufts University showed that elderly nursing home residents ranging in age from 86 to 96 dramatically increased their strength and improved their balance after just eight weeks of supervised weight training. Now studies have proved that working out with free weights or machines can help restore lost bone density, as well as reducing knee pain from arthritis and helping to keep the body sensitive to the insulin it produces and to keep sugar levels in balance.[15]

A recent study indicates that regular exercise may also reduce the risk of developing Alzheimer's disease. The study examined the long-term health habits of 373 people — 126 of them with Alzheimer's disease and 247 of them without. The patients with Alzheimer's disease had had lower levels of physical activity earlier in life.[16]

Exercise also reduces the need for medications such as antihypertensives, antidepressants and hypnotics that can alter balance and coordination and result in a fall.[17]

Types of exercise

1. Aerobic

This increases cardiovascular function and strength. Walking is a great aerobic exercise and the leg and hip bones are stimulated by the impact of your feet hitting the ground. There is, however, little or no evidence that aerobic exercise alone will increase bone density.

2. Flexibility

Stretching exercises promote flexibility, which in turn helps to prevent falls. Having strong and flexible joints also means that you are less likely to suffer joint injuries. Yoga is an excellent form of flexibility exercise. It is weight-bearing exercise and in the various yoga postures the muscles pull on the bone, stimulating further remodelling.

3. Balance training

This is exercise as in t'ai chi or other programmes specially designed to improve balance. As we age, our sense of balance becomes less, and as a consequence we are more at risk of falling.

4. Resistance or strength training

Many studies have now confirmed that strength training by using weights and high-impact exercises can build bone. As muscles contract when we lift weights, they pull on the bone they are attached to which then stimulates the bone to build in that area. For this reason is it important to practise a range of exercises that will stimulate the whole skeleton, particularly those areas at higher risk for fracture.

All four of these types are important in maintaining fitness, good health, and in preventing osteoporosis, but for exercise to be most effective in preventing or slowing bone loss, it must stress the skeleton. As long as exercise does not involve any sudden or excessive strain on the bones and it is compatible with a person's general health, then the more exercise the better from a skeletal point of view. Doing the exercises in different ways is also supposed to be good. The idea is if you can surprise the bone in the way you load it, that may be a way to continue to stimulate more bone mineralisation and bone strengthening.

A heavier load lifted fewer times is better than a lighter load lifted more often. A 1996 exercise study compared two types of strength-training regimes which differed in the number of repetitions and the weights lifted. The strength programme which involved high loads with low repetitions significantly increased bone density at the hip and forearm sites, whereas the endurance programme which featured low loads and high repetitions, had no effect.[18] Strength training is also important for maintaining muscle strength with ageing.

Weight training attempts to isolate specific muscle groups in various parts of your body — your shoulders, chest, arms, back, legs and stomach — and work them one at a time. A variety of exercises are available for each muscle group. Most experts recommend that you establish a routine that works all of the different muscle groups at least once during the course of a week. It's also advisable to change your weight training routine periodically by trying new exercises that will work the muscles in a slightly different way. The following exercises, which cover all the muscle groups, are suggested for healthy adults.[19] It is important always to learn safe lifting techniques. Ask an expert to teach you how to do them.

- Biceps curl
- Overhead press
- Wrist curl
- Reverse wrist curl
- Triceps extension
- Forearm pronation/supination
- Bench press
- Leg press
- Half squats
- Hip abduction/adduction
- Hamstring curl
- Hip flexion
- Hip extension

It is important to understand that a woman's body will respond differently to weight training than a man's will because of hormonal differences. The hormone testosterone plays a major role in muscular development. Because women have very little of this, they tend not to 'bulk up' with weight training.

How to get started

To begin, it is best to follow a routine developed by a qualified trainer. This does not mean you have to sign up with a personal trainer or join an expensive gym, although it helps tremendously to have a qualified expert demonstrate technique and form. But if you can't afford to do that, a simple trip to the library can be helpful. Many websites are also available to help you get started with your weight training programme. Fitnesslink.com has been recommended. This website provides training programmes for the beginner as well as the advanced weight lifter, and offers a variety of exercises so that you may change your routine frequently.

Miriam Nelson's book *Strong Women, Strong Bones* (Lothian Books, 2000) has excellent exercise programmes for beginners and those more advanced, which you can do at home for minimal cost. Her book subscribes very much to the osteoporosis epidemic theory and could therefore be read selectively. But it also has good nutritional advice and is an excellent tool for anyone who wants to do weight training at home. She also has a website, www.strongwomen.com, and for a fee will provide you with a personalised exercise programme.

The first word of advice on lifting weights is proceed with caution. It's essential to begin with very, very light weights — weights that are so easy to lift they seem to be flying through the air. Don't try to prove yourself. Strength comes with time and practice, and by starting out too heavy too soon, you could end up with injuries that prevent you from exercising at all.

General rules about resistance training

1. A warm-up is essential and will help prevent injury. Walking in place, stepping, or skipping for a few minutes will help get your muscles geared up for action.
2. Go slow. Start out light and lift the weights slowly, in a controlled manner.

3. Most experts recommend that you exercise larger muscle groups before smaller ones to achieve maximum benefits.

4. Use the same amount of weight in your left and right hands. Even if one side of your body seems to be stronger, you should be consistent in the amount of weights you use.

5. Don't overtrain. Take one or two days off before exercising the same muscle group a second time.

6. Follow your trainer's or workout routine's instructions about the number of times to lift each weight (repetitions), and how many sets of each exercise to do.

7. Don't forget to breathe! Keep your muscles oxidised.

8. Stretch at the completion of your workout to help avoid stiffness and injury.

Precautions

It is extremely important that anyone who undertakes strength training is properly supervised to ensure good technique, especially if they have low bone mass. Weight training may be dangerous if performed improperly or without supervision. If you already have osteoporosis, or have had a fragility fracture, it is very important that you avoid high-impact weightlifting, jumping, abrupt or explosive movements, twisting movements, and intense abdominal exercises. Individuals with high blood pressure, back problems or hernias should consult a doctor prior to engaging in a weight-training programme.

How often should you exercise?

Most exercise regimens which have shown a significant effect in slowing or preventing bone loss have been achieved by exercising for one hour, two to three times a week. This has been shown to be as effective as exercising every day.[20] It doesn't mean that you have to start at that level, you can begin by easing yourself into an exercise programme, and gradually increase the time. For elderly or sedentary people, exercise should be gradually introduced to minimise fatigue and sore muscles. It is also important to have variety in the programme and make sure that all muscle groups are being exercised. A carefully supervised progressive strength-training programme can do that.

Adding weights to the body during aerobic exercise is an excellent way to do at least two forms of exercise simultaneously. Ankle and arm weights which can be purchased cheaply can be worn for short periods during light exercise.

Summary

Exercise is the single most important strategy to maintain healthy bones. In order for exercise to be effective it must be continued throughout life. If we are immobile or inactive it will lead to bone loss. Sustained weight-bearing exercise will maintain bone formation and help prevent fracture. Older people who walk and exercise regularly have better coordination, muscle strength and flexibility — all important factors in preventing falls.

Conclusion

I N A JUST A FEW YEARS A RELATIVELY RARE DISEASE OF fragile bones has become a household word. Osteoporosis, now redefined as a measure of low bone density, is placed high on the medical agenda as a major threat to all women after menopause — despite widely varying diagnostic standards and a lack of evidence that low bone density even accurately predicts future fracture. Now frightened women demand bone density testing and take bone-sparing drugs, while children and adults alike drink milk to build strong bones believing this to be the best source of calcium. The industry giant that identified the osteoporosis 'epidemic' is the same one that simultaneously came up with the solutions of bone density testing and drug therapies. Once the calcium and dairy industries were on board, a phenomenal growth industry was formed that continues to expand unchecked worldwide.

Now drugs that slow down bone density loss are recording phenomenal sales and there is a proliferation of bone densitometry machines. It was so easy to convince us all that we were at risk for osteoporosis. How did this happen and why didn't anyone challenge the sudden emergence of the disease and the questionable claims made in the accompanying massive marketing campaigns?

In reality, journalists rushing to meet deadlines have little or no time to check or challenge information. Few claims by 'experts' are ever verified. More than half of the content of major papers like the *Wall Street Journal* has come straight off the fax machine and no changes are made before it is seen in print.[1] Sometimes the commercially driven operations the journalists work for have restrictions imposed on them by the powerful clients who advertise with them.

Medical research is now largely funded by companies interested in the results. Although many studies are no doubt objective and scientific, the companies with a vested interest in the result have been known to 'massage' the figures and conveniently suppress some of the findings.[2] The US Food and Drug Administration (FDA) the 'watchdog' of the western world, is reliant on the data supplied by the manufacturer requesting the license for their drug. The FDA doesn't independently test the drug; they rely on the information they are given.

And with less and less public funding available these days, even the universities are forced to accept funding from 'interested' parties. A significant percentage of pharmaceutical research conducted in universities in the US is reported to be funded by large corporations. It is not uncommon for drug companies to donate whole buildings and even endow professorships at the universities and hospitals where their products are tested and developed.[3]

Fortunately not everyone has been convinced. The controversy surrounding osteoporosis is evident in the medical journals. Independent researchers, international assessment agencies, even world experts in osteoporosis have been strenuously objecting to the defining of osteoporosis in terms of low bone density. They also question the statistics claiming high global incidence of fracture. But slowing the juggernaut isn't easy and challenging it can have consequences. One medical official in British Columbia who made a stand and temporarily reversed the tide of DXA machine purchasing there lost his job as a result.[4]

The medical profession is trapped. Doctors are at their most knowledgeable immediately after their training. From that time on their main source of new information is drug companies that sponsor and run conventions, 'seminars' and 'training courses', often in alluring holiday resorts, with free travel and accommodation. The speakers are mostly respected medical specialists, paid by the drug companies to talk about developments in managing the disease treated by the company's product.

Doctors are also kept up to date with new drugs by company representatives who support the efficacy of the product with research commissioned by the company. Safety is always an issue for doctors too, and working within the parameters laid down by the companies helps protect them from malpractice suits.

But the biggest problem in the end may be us — the women. Frightened by worrying statistics, images of crumbling spines and the wheelchair-bound elderly, we turn up in doctors' waiting-rooms wanting solutions. It is a brave doctor who recommends weight-bearing exercise and a change in diet to a woman bearing DXA scan results revealing low bone mineral density. All the messages we are receiving imply there is a magic bullet that will sort the problem out, that it is never too late.

So much is still not understood about osteoporosis and as it turns out, just about every aspect of bone research is a matter of hot debate. Hopefully some day it will lead to safe, effective solutions to fragility fracture. In the meantime, regular weight-bearing exercise, excellent nutrition, lowered exposure to environmental toxins and successful management of stress obviously have a large part to play. But until we have found a way not to age, then a proportion of us will inevitably suffer age-related disorders. One of these is low bone density, and in combination with other risk factors, the chance of fracture.

My undertaking to learn about osteoporosis and try to find a solution for my family took me down a fascinating path. Having previously accepted conventional wisdom regarding osteoporosis, I was stunned by the conflicting information I found in the course of my research. There still remain many unanswered questions and I do not dismiss the potential for serious problems for my son, daughter and other family members later in life. Our family history of childhood fracture and the very low bone density in some of us significantly increase our risk for fragility fracture. But at the same time, a dire prognosis is far from confirmed. Because there is naturally a wide biological variation in bone density in healthy adults, it could be that our bone strength and micro-architecture is sound, and that low bone density is normal for us and not a predictor of adult fracture.

Nor is the progression of bone health over a lifetime understood. At this point no one can say what the future holds. My parents are now in their late 70s and early 80s. It is over six years since they were diagnosed with osteoporosis in terms of low bone density and neither of them has fractured. In fact none of us have. We are all fit and well, including Camille. It is seven years since she has fractured and she leads a very active life. She attends dance classes, and exercises using Pilates techniques several times a week. (Pilates is an individually tailored exercise system focused on improving flexibility and strength for the total body.) She has even been brave enough to go back to the ski slopes and has managed to avoid injury. My son Jude, now married and living in North America, is an avid roller-blader and lover of the great Canadian outdoors.

The search is far from over. There is evidence (from hair mineral analysis) that some of our family have very low levels of boron, which could indicate some inability, possibly genetic, to absorb this trace mineral. As boron is a necessary element in the bone remodelling process, we may have a clue in this. We are pursuing it further.

It is clear that osteoporosis as defined by fragility fracture is a complex and multifactorial disease. With the exception of the very elderly and the ill, it appears it is also a rare disease. Defining osteoporosis simply as a measure of low bone density is causing unnecessary fear and leads to the massive overprescription of drugs which are potentially dangerous, and at this time, of minimal benefit.

There is a worrying lack of readily available information on osteoporosis that is not commercially motivated. It is essential that all of us are educated about the accuracy of diagnostic methods and the safety and effectiveness of any treatment before we embark upon them. The intention of this book is to help diminish the current information gap by giving a broader and lesser known perspective on the issues associated with osteoporosis. My hope is that it provides useful evidence-based information and positive direction for anyone who has been diagnosed with osteoporosis or believes they are at risk of fragility fracture.

Steps to take following a diagnosis of low bone density

The rush to measure bone density in apparently healthy women has placed many doctors in a difficult situation. What do they do when their patient brings them a DXA print-out showing that they have low bone density? Many general practitioners accept unquestioningly that a low bone density reading is a precursor to a disabling fracture and reach for the prescription pad, believing this is the best thing they can do for their patient. Chances are, however, that it is not. The following are questions that need to be asked in order to determine your actual risk for fracture. The first three questions are considered the most important.

Osteoporosis checklist:

1. What is your age?
A woman of 50 is very unlikely to have a fracture related to osteoporosis, whereas a woman of 80 years has a 15 percent

chance of breaking her hip. Therefore, your age is an important factor in deciding what the next step will be.

2. Have you had a fracture since your 40th birthday?

A personal history of low-trauma fracture is one of the most important risk factors because it demonstrates that your bones are possibly already fragile, not just that they have the potential to be. Low trauma means fracturing a bone with minimal impact.

3. Has your mother fractured her hip?

Family history is a strong determining factor, especially immediate family.

4. Do you exercise regularly?

A sedentary lifestyle can cause bone loss. Regular exercise sustains bone remodelling, and helps prevent falls in the elderly.

5. Do you smoke more than 20 cigarettes a day?

Smokers are more at risk than nonsmokers because of the tendency to have lower bone density, lower body weight, and lower oestrogen levels.

6. What do you weigh?

Low body weight is a strong predictor of fracture risk, and it is generally believed that a weight of 60 kg or more offers protection. Weight loss is to be avoided where possible as it is associated with significant BMD loss in postmenopausal women. Conversely, it is also the case that small bones automatically register lower on bone density tests even if they are not thinner, which can make small bones look more at risk than they are.

7. Have you lost height lately?

Find out if there has been height loss and how much. Loss of height can be related to compression of discs, but a loss of height of more than 3 cm usually indicates vertebral deformity.

8. Do you suffer frequently from diarrhoea?

This could be caused by problems such as celiac disease or Crohn's disease.

9. Did you have an early menopause or a surgical menopause?

This can cause a more rapid bone loss in some women.

10. Have your periods stopped for 12 months or more (other than because of pregnancy)?

Eating disorders, over-exercising and emotional trauma may all interfere with normal menstruation. This in turn can influence bone remodelling and cause reduced bone density.

11. What prescription medications are you taking?

Certain drugs like corticosteroids are associated with bone loss and increased rate of fracture. (See full list of drugs on pages 98–100).

APPENDIX II

Tests for secondary causes

If your bone density is very low (or even if your bone density is normal) and you want to eliminate other risk factors, then ask your doctor for the following tests:

1. If you have lost height and if your DXA scan shows low BMD in the spine then a lateral spine X-ray will determine whether there has been any compression fracturing.

2. Blood (serum) vitamin D and calcium levels, and a lactose tolerance test.

3. A thyroid test — especially if there is a family history of hyperthyroidism.

4. A 24-hour calcium/urine test will measure how much calcium is being lost in the urine. If there are high levels of calcium in the urine then you need to see a specialist.

5. Measure more than one bone site. It is possible that there can be some inaccuracies with DXA scanning, particularly if you have already had a spinal fracture which has caused some compression in your vertebrae. This can make your bones seem denser than they are. Sometimes we are not aware that we have had a fracture of the vertebrae as they can be painless, so measuring the hip as well can give a more accurate reading.

6. A bone marker urine test will give some idea of what rate of bone breakdown or resorption of bone is going on by measuring the breakdown products of collagen. It is normally quite high postmenopausally, but repeat testing every 3–6 months will indicate whether changes are occurring. The tests to request are Dpd or deoxypyridinoline and NTx or N-telopeptide which measure bone breakdown or resorption, and ALP or bone alkaline phosphatase which measures bone formation.

7. Celiac disease. There are three useful antibody blood tests which, if all three come back positive, indicate there is a very high chance that you have celiac disease. They are: endomysial, reticulin (IgA), and gliadin (IgG and IgA).

8. If you are male, then serum testosterone levels could also be measured.

9. Have blood levels of magnesium, zinc, manganese, boron and other trace minerals tested.

10. Hair mineral analysis is a useful way of finding out whether you have mineral deficiencies which may affect bone health. These days sophisticated methods of analysis can give accurate readings.

NOTES

INTRODUCTION

1 Cardon, L.R. et al. 'Evidence for
   a major gene for bone mineral
   density in idiopathic osteoporotic
   families'. *Journal of Bone and
   Mineral Research* 2000;
   15(60):1132–1137.

CHAPTER ONE
*The epidemic — is the emperor
wearing clothes?*

1 National Osteoporosis
   Foundation (US).
   http://www.nof.org/

2 http://www.nof.org/news/
   pressreleases/prevmo_2001.html

3 Genant, H.K. et al. Interim
   report and recommendations of
   the World Health Organisation
   Task-force for osteoporosis.

Osteoporosis International 1999;
10:259–264.

4 'Clinical Management Guidelines
   for Osteoporosis in Hong Kong'.
   Hong Kong Medical Journal
   1998; 4:423–431.

5 International Osteoporosis
   Foundation website. http://
   www.osteofound.org/
   press_centre/
   scrip_magazine.html

6 Ahmed, A.I.H. et al. 'Screening
   for osteopenia and osteoporosis:
   Do the accepted normal ranges
   lead to overdiagnosis?'
   Osteoporosis International 1997;
   7:432–438.

7 Pors Nielsen, S. 'The fallacy of
   BMD: A critical review of the
   diagnostic use of dual X-ray
   absorptiometry'.

Clinical Rheumatology 2000;
19(3):174–183

8   Heaney, R.P. 'Sources of bone
    fragility'. *Osteoporosis
    International* 2000;
    Suppl.2:S43–46.

9   Weinsier, R.L. 'Dairy foods and
    bone health: Examination of the
    evidence'. *American Journal of
    Clinical Nutrition* 2000;
    72:681–689.

10 Lopez, J.M. et al. 'Bone turnover
    and density in healthy women
    during breastfeeding and after
    weaning'. *Osteoporosis
    International* 1996; 6:153–159.

11 Rubin, S.M., Cummings, S.R.
    'Results of bone densitometry
    affect women's decisions about
    taking measures to prevent
    fractures'. *Annals of Internal
    Medicine* 1992;
    116(12 Pt1):990–995.

12 Marci, C.D., Viechnicki, M.B.
    and Greenspan, S.L. 'Bone
    mineral densitometry
    substantially influences health-
    related behaviors of
    postmenopausal women'.
    Calcified Tissue International
    2000 Feb; 66(2):113–118.

13 Dequeker, J. et al. 'Hip fracture
    and osteoporosis in a XIIth
    Dynasty female skeleton from
    Lisht, Upper Egypt'. *Journal of
    Bone and Mineral Research* 1997;
    12(6):881–888.

14 'Bone mineral testing: Does the
    evidence support its selective use

in well women?' British Columbia
Office of Health Technology
Assessment, December 1997.
www.chspr.ubc.ca

15 http://washingtonpost.com/wp-
    dyn/articles/A14106–
    2000Sep25.html

16 Papanikolaw, J. 'Hormone
    replacement therapy set for
    growth in developed nations'.
    Chemical Market Reporter
    December 20 1999. http://
    www.findarticles.com

17 Kazanjian, A., Green, C. and
    Bassett, K. 'Normal bone mass,
    ageing bodies, marketing of fear:
    Bone mineral density screening
    of well women'. British Columbia
    Office of Health Technology
    Assessment September 1998.
    www.chspr.ubc.ca

18 'Bone mineral testing: Does the
    evidence support its selective use
    in well women?' ibid.

19 Genant, H.K. et al. Interim
    Report and Recommendations of
    the WHO Task-Force for
    Osteoporosis. *Osteoporosis
    International* 1999; 19:259–264.

20 Ott, Susan, MD. Personal
    correspondence with the author,
    April 3 2001.

21 Kazanjian, A. et al. 'Bone mineral
    testing in social context'.
    *International Journal of
    Technology Assessment in Health
    Care* 1999; 15(4):679–685.

22 Keating, N.L. et al. 'Use of
    hormone replacement by

postmenopausal women in the United States'. *Ann Intern Med* 1999; 130(7):545–553.

23 WHO Geneva 1994. 'Assessment of fracture risk and its application to screening for postmenopausal osteoporosis'. WHO Technical Report Series 843.

24 Ringertz, H. et al. 'Bone density measurement: A systematic review'. A report from SBU, the Swedish Council on Technology Assessment in Health Care. *Journal of Internal Medicine* 1997; 241(Suppl.739):i–iii,1–60.

25 Dewar, Elaine. 'Breaking news: blowing the whistle on osteoporosis'. *Homemakers* October 1998; 57–70.

26 Davis, J.W. et al. 'The peak bone mass of Hawaiian, Filipino, Japanese, and white women living in Hawaii'. *Calcif Tissue Int* 1994; 55:249–52.

27 Melton, L.J. III et al. 'Effects of body size and skeletal site on the estimated prevalence of osteoporosis in women and men'. *Osteoporosis International* 2000; 11:977–983.

28 *Medical Device & Diagnostic Industry Magazine*. November 1995. http://www.devicelink.com/mddi/archive/95/11/004.html

29 'Bone mineral testing: Does the evidence support its selective use in well women?' ibid.

30 Pors Neilsen, S. ibid.

31 Coney, S. *The Menopause Industry*. Penguin Books NZ 1992, p. 107.

32 Law, M.R. et al. 'Strategies for prevention of osteoporosis and hip fracture'. *British Medical Journal* 1991; 303:453–459.

33 Coney, S. ibid.

34 http://osteoporosis.org.nz/links.html

35 'Osteoporosis and bone physiology'. The website of Susan Ott MD, Associate Professor of Medicine at the University of Washington. http://courses.washington.edu/bonephys/

36 http://www.nof.org/

37 Tenenhouse, A. et al. 'Estimation of the prevalence of low bone density in Canadian women and men using a population-specific DXA reference standard: The Canadian Multicentre Osteoporosis Study (CaMos)'. *Osteoporosis International* 2000; 11:897–904.

38 Looker, A.C. et al. 'Prevalence of low femoral density in older US women from National Health and Nutrition Examination Survey III (NHANES III), conducted between 1988 and 1991'. *J Bone Min Res* 1995; 10:796–802.

39 http://www.osteofound.org/

40 www.nos.org.uk

41 http://www.osteofound.org/member_societies/australia2.html

42 *New Zealand Herald*. Monday April 23, 2001.

43 Ott, Susan, MD. Correspondence with the author. November 2000.

44 Heaney, R.P. 'Sources of Bone Fragility'. *Osteoporosis International* 2000; Suppl.2:S43–46.

45 'Bone mineral testing: Does the evidence support its selective use in well women?' ibid.

46 Kazanjian, A. et al. 'BMD testing in social context'. *International Journal of Technology Assessment in Health Care* 1999; 15(4):679–685.

47 'Bone mineral testing: Does the evidence support its selective use in well women?' ibid.

48 Walker, A. 'Osteoporosis and calcium deficiency'. *Am J Clin Nutr* 1965; 16:327–336.

49 Starfield, B. 'Is US health really the best in the world?' *Journal of the American Medical Association* 2000; 284(4):483–485.

CHAPTER TWO
Bone and bone metabolism

1 Calbet, J.A.L. et al. 'High bone mineral density in male élite professional volleyball players'. *Osteoporosis International* 1999; 10:468–474.

2 Heaney, R.P. et al. 'Peak bone mass'. *Osteoporosis International* 2000; 11:985–1009.

3 Dewar, Elaine. 'Breaking News – blowing the whistle on osteoporosis'. *Homemakers* (Canada) October 1998.

CHAPTER THREE
Fractures — the facts

1 Cited in 'Osteoporosis and bone physiology'. The website of Susan Ott MD, Associate Professor of Medicine at the University of Washington. http://courses.washington.edu/bonephys/

2 Pors Neilsen, S. 'The fallacy of BMD: A critical review of the diagnostic use of Dual X-ray Absorptiometry'. *Clinical Rheumatology* 2000; 19(3):174–183.

3 Myers, E.R. et al. 'Geometric variables from DXA of the radius predict forearm fracture load in vitro'. *Calcified Tissue International* 1993; 52:199–204.

4 Doherty D. et al. 'Lifetime and five-year age-specific risks of first and subsequent osteoporotic fractures in postmenopausal women'. *Osteoporosis International* 2001; 12:16–23.

5 Heaney, R.P. 'Bone mass, fragility and the decision to treat' (Editorial). *Journal of the American Medical Association* 1998; 280(24):2119–2120.

6 Ott, Susan MD. 'Osteoporosis and bone physiology'. ibid.

7 Frost, H.M. 'Personal experience in managing acute compression fractures, their aftermath, and the bone pain syndrome in osteoporosis'. *Osteoporosis International* 1998; 8:13–15.

8 Bennell, K. et al. 'The role of physiotherapy in the prevention and treatment of osteoporosis'. *Manual Therapy* 2000; 5(4):198–213.

9 Ott, Susan MD. Correspondence with the author. March 4 2001.

10 Lunt, M. et al. 'Population-based geographic variations in DXA bone density in Europe: The EVOS study'. *Osteoporosis International* 1997; 7:175–189.

11 Ettinger, B. Correspondence with the author, 23 April 2001.

12 http://www.studd.co.uk/osteoporosis.html

13 Burger, H., van Daele, P.L.A., Grashuis, K. et al. 'Vertebral deformities and functional impairment in men and women'. *Journal of Bone and Mineral Research* 1997; 12:152–157.

14 Jackson, S.A., Tenenhouse, A., Robertson, L. and the CaMos Study group. 'Vertebral fracture definition from population-based data: preliminary results from the Canadian multicentre osteoporosis study (CaMos)'. *Osteoporosis International* 2000; 11:680–687.

15 Ott, Susan MD. 'Osteoporosis and bone physiology'. ibid.

16 'Osteoporosis Prevention, Diagnosis, and Therapy'. US National Institute of Health (NIH) Consensus Statement 2000; March 27–29; 17(1):1–36.

17 Holmes, J. et al. 'Psychiatric assessment advised for patients with hip fracture'. *The Lancet* 2001; 357:1264.

18 'Osteoporosis Prevention, Diagnosis, and Therapy'. (NIH) Consensus Statement. ibid.

19 Hegsted, D.M., 'Calcium and osteoporosis'. *Journal of Nutrition* 1986; 116:2316–2319.

20 Norton, R. et al. 'Hip fracture incidence among older people in Auckland'. *New Zealand Medical Journal* 1995; 108:426–428.

21 Xu, Ling. et al. 'Very low rates of hip fracture in Beijing, People's Republic of China'. The Beijing Osteoporosis Project, *American Journal of Epidemiology* 1996; 144:901–907.

22 Hayes, W.C. et al. 'Etiology and prevention of age-related hip fractures'. *Bone* 1996; 18:77S–86S.

23 Ott, Susan MD. Correspondence with the author, 16 October 2000.

24 Mautalen, C.A. et al. 'Are the etiologies of cervical and trochanteric hip fractures different?' *Bone* 1996; 18:133S–137S.

25 Cummings, S.R. et al. 'Racial differences in hip axis length might explain racial differences in rates of hip fracture'. *Osteoporosis International* 1994; 4:226–229.

26 'Padded clothing prevents life-threatening hip fractures'. *ADVANCE for Physical*

Therapists and PT Assistants,
November 2, 2000.

CHAPTER FOUR
Doubtful diagnoses

1 Ott, Susan MD. 'Osteoporosis and bone physiology'. http://courses.washington.edu/bonephys

2 'Bone mineral testing: Does the evidence support its selective use in well women?' British Columbia Office of Health Technology Assessment, December 1997. www.chspr.ubc.ca

3 ibid.

4 Genant, H.K. et al. Interim Report and Recommendations of the WHO Task-force for Osteoporosis. *Osteoporosis International* 1999; 10:259–264.

5 Heaney, R.P. 'Sources of bone fragility'. *Osteoporosis International* 2000; Suppl.2:S43–46.

6 Ott, Susan MD. Correspondence with the author. November 2000.

7 Ott, Susan MD. ibid.

8 Karlsson, M.K. et al. 'Bone mineral normative data in Malmo, Swedena; Comparison with reference data and hip fracture incidence in other ethnic groups'. *Acta Orthopaedica Scandinavica* 1993; 64(2):168–172. (Cited in BCHOTA Review. www.chspr.ubc.ca)

9 Law, M.R. et al. 'Strategies for prevention of osteoporosis and hip fracture'. *British Medical Journal* 1991; 303:453–459.

10 ibid.

11 Melton, L.J. III et al. 'Effects of body size and skeletal site on the estimated prevalence of osteoporosis in women and men'. *Osteoporosis International* 2000; 11:977–983.

12 Tenenhouse, A. Correspondence with the author. November 20 2000.

13 Kanis, J.A. et al. 'An update on the diagnosis and assessment of osteoporosis with densitometry'. Position Paper. *Osteoporosis International* 2000; 11:192–202.

14 Pors Nielson, S. 'The fallacy of BMD: A critical review of the diagnostic use of dual X-ray absorptiometry'. *Clinical Rheumatology* 2000; 19:174–183.

15 ibid.

16 'Bone mineral testing: Does the evidence support its selective use in well women?' ibid.

17 Dewar, Elaine. 'Breaking news: Blowing the whistle on the osteoporosis epidemic'. *Homemakers* (Canada) October 1998; pp. 57–70.

18 Law, M.R. et al. ibid.

19 Bachrach, L.K. 'Acquisition of optimal bone mass in childhood and adolescence'. *Trends in Endocrinology and Metabolism* January–February 2001; 12(1):22–28.

20 'Bone mineral testing: Does the

evidence support its selective use in well women?' ibid.

21 ibid.

22 Kanis, J.A. et al. ibid.

23 'Bone mineral testing: Does the evidence support its selective use in well women?' ibid.

24 Looker, A.C. et al. 'Prevalence of low femoral bone density in older us women from NHANES III'. *Journal of Bone and Mineral Research* 1995; 10(5):796–802.

25 Kanis, J.A. and Gluer, C.-C., ibid.

26 Tenenhouse, A. et al. 'Estimation of the prevalence of low bone density in Canadian women and men using a population-specific DXA reference standard: The Canadian Multicentre Osteoporosis Study (CaMos)'. *Osteoporosis International* 2000; 11:897–904.

27 The CaMos website: http://www.camos.org/

28 Gurlek, A. et al. 'Inappropriate reference range for peak bone mineral density in dual-energy X-ray absorptiometry: Implications for the interpretation of T-scores'. *Osteoporosis International* 2000; 11(9):809–813.

29 Ahmed, A.I.H. et al. 'Screening for osteopenia and osteoporosis: Do the accepted normal ranges lead to overdiagnosis?' *Osteoporosis International* 1997; 7:432–438.

30 Simmons, A. et al. 'Dual energy X-ray absorptiometry normal reference range use within the UK and the effect of different normal ranges on the assessment of bone density'. *British Journal of Radiology* 1995; 68(812):903–909.

31 Ahmed, A.I.H. ibid.

32 Pors Nielsen, S. ibid.

33 Delmas, P.D. 'Do we need to change the WHO definition of osteoporosis?' *Osteoporosis International* 2000; 11:189–191.

34 'Bone mineral testing: Does the evidence support its selective use in well women?' ibid.

35 Kanis, J.A. 'Diagnosis of osteoporosis'. *Osteoporosis International* 1997; 7 Suppl.3:S108–116.

36 Conversation between the author and a representative of Norland International. March 2001.

37 Elliot, J.R. et al. 'Effects of age and sex on bone density at the hip and spine in a normal Caucasian New Zealand population'. *New Zealand Medical Journal* 1990; 103:33–36.

38 Kazanjian, A. et al. 'Bone mineral testing in social context'. *International Journal of Technology Assessment in Health Care* 1999; 15:679–685.

39 Le Lorier, J. et al. 'Older women may not use HRT long enough to benefit'. *Journal of Obstetrics and Gynecology* 2001; 97:97–100.

40 Marci, C.D. et al. 'Bone mineral densitometry substantially

influences health-related behaviors of postmenopausal women'. *Calcified Tissue International* February 2000; 66(2):113–118.

41 Varney, L.F. et al. 'Classification of osteoporosis and osteopenia in postmenopausal women is dependent on site-specific analysis'. *Journal of Clinical Densitometry* 1999; 2:275–283.

42 ibid.

43 'Bone mineral testing: Does the evidence support its selective use in well women?' ibid.

44 Homick, J. and Bailey, D. Bone density measurement: A health technology report, 1999. Alberta Heritage Foundation for Medical Research.

45 University of Newcastle Osteoporosis Study Group. Meta-analysis of interventions for prevention and treatment of post-menopausal osteoporosis and fracture. Final report: Estrogen treatment, results of published trials and epidemiological studies, assessment of study quality and public health implications. Warratah, Australia: University of Newcastle, 1995. (Cited in BCOHTA Review www.chspr.ubc.ca)

46 'Bone mineral testing: Does the evidence support its selective use in well women?' ibid.

47 Ringertz, H. et al. 'Bone density measurement: A systematic review'. A report from SBU, the Swedish Council on Technology Assessment in Health Care. *Journal of Internal Medicine* 1997; 241(Suppl.)739:i–iii, 1–60.

48 Hailey, D. et al. INAHTA project on the effectiveness of density measurement and associated treatments for prevention of fractures. Statement of findings. September 1996. http://www.ahfmr.ab.ca/hta/hta-publications/joint/bdm.stmt.shtml

49 ibid.

50 Bassett, Ken. 'On trying to stop the measurement of bone density to sell drugs: A tribute to a friend'. *Tales from other drug wars*. Papers from the 12th Annual Health Policy Conference, held in Vancouver, British Columbia, November 26, 1999. ISBN 0–88865–240–242.

51 'Bone mineral testing: Does the evidence support its selective use in well women?' ibid.

52 Homick, J. and Bailey, D. ibid.

53 Effectiveness bulletin from the University of Leeds. 'A Review: Bandolier evidence-based health care'. http://www.jr2.ox.ac.uk/bandolier/band3/b3–4.html

CHAPTER FIVE
Risk factors for osteoporosis

1 'Bone mineral testing: Does the evidence support its selective use in well women?' British Columbia

Office of Health Technology Assessment, December 1997. www.chspr.ubc.ca

2 Tannirandorn, P., Epstein, S. 'Drug-induced bone loss'. *Osteoporosis International* 2000; 11:637–659.

3 'Osteoporosis Prevention, Diagnosis, and Therapy'. US National Institute of Health (NIH) Consensus Statement 2000; March 27–29; 17(1):1–36.

4 ibid.

5 ibid.

6 ibid.

7 Orwoll, E.S. 'Determinants of bone mineral density in older men'. *Osteoporosis International* 2000; 11:815–821.

8 Homick, J., Bailey, D. 'Bone density measurement: A health technology report'. Alberta Heritage Foundation for Medical Research. http:/www.ahfmr.ab.ca/hta/hta publicat...reports/bonedensity99/bonedensity.shtml

9 Cummings, S.R. et al. 'Risk factors for hip fracture in white women'. *New England Journal of Medicine* 1995; 332(12):767–774.

10 ibid.

11 Cumming, R.G., Klineberg, R.J., 'Case-control study of risk factors for hip fracture in the elderly'. *American Journal of Epidemiology* 1994; 139:493–503.

12 Tannirandorn, P., Epstein, S. ibid.

13 Sategna-Guidetti, C. et al. 'The effects of 1-year gluten withdrawal on bone mass, bone metabolism and nutritional status in newly-diagnosed adult coeliac disease patients'. *Alimentary Pharmacology and Therapeutics* 2000 January; 14(1):35–43.

14 Mora, S. et al. 'Reversal of low bone density with a gluten-free diet in children and adolescents with celiac disease'. *American Journal of Clinical Nutrition* 1998; 67(3):477–481.

15 Chapuy, M.C. et al. 'Vitamin D3 and calcium to prevent hip fractures in elderly women'. *NEJM* 1992; 327:1637–1642.

16 Glerup, H. et al. 'Commonly recommended daily intake of Vitamin D is not sufficient if sunlight exposure is limited'. *Journal of Internal Medicine* 2000; 247(2):260–268.

17 From *Medscape News* May 8, 2001. Garg, R. et al. 'Elderly Lack Adequate Levels of Vitamin D'. Posted at the American Association of Clinical Endocrinologists 10th Annual Meeting, held in San Antonio, Texas.

18 Bennell, K. et al. 'The role of physiotherapy in the prevention and treatment of osteoporosis'. *Manual Therapy* 2000; 5(4):198–213.

19 Robertson, M.C. et al. 'Effectiveness and economic evaluation of a nurse-delivered home exercise programme to

prevent falls. 2: A controlled trial in multiple centres'. *British Medical Journal* 2001; 322:701–704.

20 Cadarette, S.M. et al. 'Development and validation of the osteoporosis risk assessment instrument to facilitate selection of women for bone densitometry. *Canadian Medical Association Journal* 2000; 162(9):1289–1294.

21 Robinson, E. 'Use of hormone replacement therapy to reduce the risk of osteopenia in adolescent girls with anorexia nervosa'. *Journal of Adolescent Health* 2000 May; 26(5):343–348.

22 ibid.

23 ibid.

24 Tannirandorn, P., Epstein, S. ibid.

25 ibid.

26 Cooper, C. et al. 'Corticosteroid Treatment Increased Risk Of Vertebral Fracture'. Presented at the meeting of the American Society for Bone and Mineral Research and the International Bone and Mineral Society. San Francisco, December 14, 1998.

27 Tannirandorn, P., Epstein, S. ibid.

28 ibid.

29 ibid.

30 ibid.

31 ibid.

32 Beard, J. et al. '1,1,1–Trichloro–2,2–bis (p-Chlorophenyl)-Ethane (DDT) and reduced bone mineral density'. *Archives of Environmental Health* 2000; 55(3):177–180.

33 Glynn, A.W. et al. 'Organochlorines and bone mineral density in Swedish men from the general population'. *Osteoporosis International* 2000; 11:1036–1042.

34 Colborn, Theo, et al. *Our Stolen Future*. Abacus 1997.

35 Cancer Prevention Coalition. Extract from their Consumer Right-to-Know Resolution presented to the UN Food and Agricultural Organisation Global Food Summit, Rome, 1996.

36 Wyshak, G. 'Consumption of carbonated drinks by teenage girls associated with bone fractures'. *Archives of Pediatrics and Adolescent Medicine* 2000; 154:542–543, 610–613.

37 Gaby, A. *Preventing and Reversing Osteoporosis*. Prima Health 1994.

38 Eppley, K. et al. 'Differential effects of relaxation techniques on trait anxiety'. *Journal of Clinical Psychology* 1989; 45:957–974.

39 Zhiping, Huang, Himes, J. and McGovern, P. 'Nutrition and subsequent hip fracture risk among a national cohort of white women'. *Am J Epidemiol* 1996; 144:124–134.

40 National Institutes of Health Osteoporosis and Related Bone Diseases National Resource

Centre. http://www.osteo.org/osteo.html

41 Mazess, R. et al. 'Bone density in premenopausal women: Effects of age, dietary intake, physical activity, smoking and birth control pills'. *Am J Clin Nutr* 1991; 53:132–142.

42 Baron, J. 'Current smoking increases risk of hip fracture in postmenopausal women'. *Archives of Internal Medicine* 2001; 161:983–988.

43 Tannirandorn, P., Epstein, S. ibid.

44 Baudoin, C. et al. 'Moderate alcohol consumption linked to increased bone mass in elderly women'. *Am J Epidemiol* 2000; 151:773–780.

45 Gilsanz, V. 'Differential effect of race on the axial and appendicular skeletons of children'. *Journal of Clinical Endocrinology and Metabolism* 1998 May; 83(5):1420–1427.

46 Gouling, A. et al. 'Bone mineral density in girls with forearm fractures'. *Journal of Bone and Mineral Research* 1998; 13:143–148.

47 Bachrach, L.K.J. 'Dual energy X-ray absorptiometry (DEXA) measurements of bone density and body composition: Promise and pitfalls'. *Journal of Pediatric Endocrinology and Metabolism* 2000 September; 13(Suppl.2):983–988.

CHAPTER SIX
Treatments for osteoporosis — introduction

1 Heaney, R. 'Bone mass, bone fragility and the decision to treat'. *JAMA* 1998; 280(24):2119–2120.

2 Riggs, L.B., Hodgson, S.F., O'Fallon, M. et al. 'Effect of fluoride treatment on the fracture rate of postmenopausal women with osteoporosis'. *NEJM* 1990; 322:802–809.

CHAPTER SEVEN
Hormone replacement therapy

1 Ahlgrimm, Marla. *The HRT Solution*. Avery 1999.

2 New Zealand Guidelines Group. 'The appropriate prescribing of hormone replacement therapy'. May 2001. www.nzgg.org.nz

3 Posthuma, W.F. et al. 'Cardioprotective effect of hormone replacement therapy in postmenopausal women: Is the evidence biased?' *British Medical Journal* 1994; 308:1268–1269.

4 Hulley, S. et al. 'Randomized trial of estrogen plus progestin for secondary prevention of coronary heart disease in postmenopausal women'. *Journal of the American Medical Association* 1998; 280:695–713.

5 Schairer, C. et al. 'Menopausal estrogen and estrogen-progestin replacement therapy and breast cancer risk. *JAMA* 2000; 238:485–491.

6 Collaborative Group on Hormonal Factors in Breast Cancer. 'Breast cancer and hormone replacement therapy: Collaborative reanalysis of data from 51 epidemiological studies of 52705 women with breast cancer and 108411 women without breast cancer'. *The Lancet* 1997; 350:1047–1059.

7 New Zealand Guidelines Group. ibid.

8 Hormone Replacement Therapy Fact Sheet and Women's Health Initiative (WHI) HRT Update. www.nhlbi.nih.gov/whi/hrt.htm

9 Papanikolaw, J. 'Hormone Replacement Therapy set for growth in developed nations'. *Chemical Market Reporter* December 20, 1999. http://www.findarticles.com

10 Keating, N.L. et al. 'Use of hormone replacement by postmenopausal women in the United States'. *Annals of Internal Medicine* 1999; 130(7):545–553.

11 Cummings, S.R., Browner, W.S., Bauer, D., et al. 'Endogenous hormones and the risk of hip and vertebral fractures among older women'. *New England Journal of Medicine* 1998; 339:733–738.

12 Sellmann, S. 'Osteoporosis – the Myths'. *Nexus* magazine 1998; 5(6). http://www.nexusmagazine.com/Osteoporosis.html

13 Riggs, B. and Melton, L.

'Involutional osteoporosis'. *NEJM* 1986; 26:1676–1686.

14 Riggs, B. and Melton, L. ibid.

15 Greendale, G.A. et al. 'How many women lose bone mineral density while taking hormone replacement therapy?' Results from the PEPI trial. *Archives of Internal Medicine* 2000; 160:3065–3071.

16 'Bone Mineral Testing: Does the evidence support its selective use in well women?' B.C. Office of Health Technology Assessment, December 1997. www.chspr.ubc.ca

17 Riggs, B. and Melton, L. ibid.

18 New Zealand Guidelines Group. ibid.

19 Quoted in *Health* May 31, 2001. http://www.idf50.co.uk/menopausejanet.htm

20 Komulainen, M. et al. 'Identification of early postmenopausal women with no bone response to HRT: Results of a five-year clinical trial'. *Osteoporosis International* 2000; 11(3):211–218.

21 Greendale, G.A. et al. ibid.

22 Le Lorier, J. et al. 'Older women may not use HRT long enough to benefit'. *Journal of Obstetrics and Gynecology* 2001; 97:97–100.

23 New Zealand Guidelines Group. ibid.

24 Ettinger, B. 'The waning effect of postmenopausal estrogen therapy on osteoporosis'. *NEJM* 1993; 329(16):1192–1193.

25 Colditz, G.A. 'Cumulative risk of breast cancer to age 70 years according to risk factor status: Data from the nurses' health study'. *American Journal of Epidemiology* 2000; 152:950–964.

26 Collaborative Group on Hormonal Factors in Breast Cancer. 'Breast cancer and hormone replacement therapy: Collaborative reanalysis of data from 51 epidemiological studies of 52705 women with breast cancer and 108411 women without breast cancer'. *The Lancet* 1997; 350:1047–1059.

27 Persson, I. et al. 'Risks of breast and endometrial cancer after estrogen and progestin replacement'. *Cancer Causes Control* 1998; 19:61–109.

28 Schairer, C. et al. ibid.

29 Willet, W.C. et al. 'Perimenopausal estrogens — opposed, unopposed, or none of the above' (Editorial). *JAMA* 2000; 238:534–535.

30 Tavani, A. et al. 'The adverse effects of hormone replacement therapy'. *Drugs & Aging* 1999; 14(5):347–357.

31 Kavanagh, A.M. et al. 'Hormone replacement therapy and accuracy of mammographic screening'. *The Lancet* 2000; 355:270–274.

32 Smith, W.A. et al. 'Alcohol and breast cancer in women: A pooled analysis of cohort studies'. Department of Nutrition, Harvard School of Public Health, Boston, Mass. 02115, USA. *JAMA* 1998 February; 279(7):535–540.

33 Rodriguez, C. et al. 'Estrogen replacement therapy and ovarian cancer mortality in a large prospective study of US women'. *JAMA* 2001; 285(11):1460–1465.

34 New Zealand Guidelines Group. ibid.

35 Hulley, S., Grady, D., Bush, T. et al. 'Randomized trial of estrogen plus progestin for secondary prevention of coronary heart disease in postmenopausal women'. *JAMA* 1998; 280:605–613.

36 Grodstein, F. et al. 'A prospective observational study of postmenopausal hormone therapy and primary prevention of cardiovascular disease'. *Ann Intern Med* 2000;133:933–941.

37 Grady, D. and Hulley, B. 'Hormones to prevent coronary heart disease in women'. *Ann Intern Med* 2000; 133:999–1001.

38 Hormone Replacement Therapy Fact Sheet and WHI HRT Update. www.nhlbi.nih.gov/whi/hrt-en.htm

39 ibid.

40 Grady, D. and Hulley, S. 'Hormones to prevent coronary disease in women'. *Ann Intern Med* 2000; 133(12):999–1001.

41 Meier, C.R. et al.

'Postmenopausal estrogen replacement therapy and the risk of developing lupus erythematosus or discoid lupus'. *Journal of Rheumatology* 1998; 25(8):1515–1519.

42 New Zealand Guidelines Group. ibid.

43 Barr, G.R., Harvard Medical School. Reporting to the annual meeting of American College of Chest Physicians. October 26, 2000.

44 Law, M.R. et al. 'Strategies for prevention of osteoporosis and hip fracture'. *British Medical Journal* 1991; 303:435–439.

45 Hulley, S., Grady, D., Bush, T. et al. 'Randomized trial of estrogen plus progestin for secondary prevention of heart disease in postmenopausal women'. *JAMA* 1998; 280:605–641.

46 Komulainen, M.H. 'HRT and Vitamin D in prevention of non-vertebral fractures in postmenopausal women'. *Maturitas* 1998; 31:45–54.

47 Lufkin, E.G. et al. 'Treatment of postmenopausal osteoporosis with transdermal estrogen'. *Ann Intern Med* 1992; 117:1–9.

48 Papapoulos, S.E. 'Pharmacologic management of osteoporosis; Methodological issues and results of intervention studies'. Medscape CME, Womens Health Treatment Updates 2000.

49 Pors Nielson, S. 'The fallacy of BMD: A critical review of the diagnostic use of dual X-ray absorptiometry'. *Clinical Rheumatology* 2000; 19:174–183.

50 Dr Suzanne C. Ho reporting at the Third Annual Scientific Meeting of the Hong Kong Epidemiological Association. January 2001.

51 Lieberman, S. 'A review of the effectiveness of *cimicifuga racemosa* (black cohosh) for the symptoms of menopause'. *Journal of Women's Health* 1998; 7(5):525–529.

52 McLaren-Howard, J., Grant, E. and Davies, S. 'Hormone Replacement Therapy and osteoporosis: Bone enzymes and nutrient imbalances'. *Journal of Nutritional and Environmental Medicine* 1998; 8:129–138.

53 Torgeson, D.J. and Bell-Syer, S.E. 'Hormone replacement therapy and prevention of nonvertebral fractures: a meta-analysis of randomized trials'. *JAMA* 2001; 285(22)2891–2897.

54 Grady, D. and Cummings, S.R. 'Postmenopausal hormone replacement therapy for prevention of fractures. How good is the evidence?' *JAMA* 2001; 285(22) 2090–2100.

CHAPTER EIGHT
Bisphosphonates and other treatments

1 Susan Ott. Correspondence with

the author, November 22, 2000.

2 Susan Ott website: http://courses.washington.edu/bonephys/

3 Mashiba, T. et al. 'Suppressed bone turnover by bisphosphonates increases microdamage accumulation and reduces some biomechanical properties in dog rib'. *Journal of Bone and Mineral Research* 2000; 15:613–620.

4 Graham, D.Y. et al. 'Alendronate and naproxen are synergistic for development of gastric ulcers'. *Archives of Internal Medicine* January 8, 2001; 161:107–110.

5 Tannirandorn, P. and Epstein, S. 'Drug-induced bone loss'. *Osteoporosis International* 2000; 11:637–659.

6 Cummings, S.R. et al. 'Effect of alendronate on risk of fracture in women with low bone density but without vertebral fractures'. *Journal of the American Medical Association* 1998; 280(24): 1077–2082.

7 *Therapeutics Letter* Issue 20, July–August 1997. http://www.interchg.ubc.ca/jauca/pages/letter20.htm#alendronate

8 Heaney, R. 'Bone mass, bone fragility and the decision to treat'. *JAMA* 1998; 280(24):2119–2120.

9 *Therapeutics Letter* ibid.

10 Merck Annual Report 2000. http://www.anrpt2000.com/

11 Stelfox, H.T. et al. 'Conflict of interest in the debate over calcium channel agonists'. *New England Journal of Medicine* 1998; 338:101–106.

12 McClung, M.R. et al. 'Effect of risedronate on the risk of hip fracture in elderly women'. Hip Intervention Program Study Group. *NEJM* February 1, 2001; 344(5):333–340.

13 'Drug ads may not always tell the whole story'. The *Georgia Straight* (Vancouver's News & Entertainment Weekly) December, 1999: p. 31.

14 Lovell-Smith, David. *Perfect Blood Pressure Naturally*. Penguin Books NZ 2001: pp. 91–92.

15 Papanikolaw, Jim. 'Hormone Replacement Therapy set for growth in developed nations. *Chemical Market Reporter* December 20, 1999. http://www.findarticles.com

16 Ettinger, B. et al. 'Reduction of vertebral fracture risk in postmenopausal women with osteoporosis treated with raloxifene'. *JAMA* 1999; 282:637–645.

17 'Lilly's TV ad overstates Evista's osteoporosis benefits FDA claims.' Reuters Health. September 27, 2000. Medscape—Women's Health October 2000.

18 Mintzes, Barbara. 'The truth, the half truth, and nothing like the

truth. Regulation of drug promotion in Canada'. *Tales from other drug wars*. Papers from the 12th Annual Health Policy Conference. Vancouver, B.C., November 26, 1999. ISBN 0–88865–240–2.

19 'Postmenopausal osteoporosis: Optimum time to start therapy unclear'. *Drugs & Therapy Perspectives* 1997; 10(7):8–12.

20 Cranney, A. et al. 'Calcitonin for preventing and treating corticosteroid-induced osteoporosis (Cochrane Review)'. *The Cochrane Library*, Issue 2, 2001.

21 http://courses.washington.edu/ bonephys/

22 Danielson, M.D. et al. 'Hip fractures and fluoridation in Utah's elderly population'. *JAMA* 1992; 268:746–748.

23 Jacqmin-Gadda, H. et al. 'Fluorine concentrations in drinking water and fracture in the elderly' (letter). *JAMA* 1995; 273:775–776.

24 Whitfield, J. 'The parathyroid hormones: Bone forming agents for treatment of osteoporosis'. Medscape — Women's Health 5(5) 2000. http:// www.medscape.com

25 http:// womenshealth.medscape.com/ reuters/prof (published in *NEJM* 2001; 344:1434–1441.)

26 Wuster, C. et al. 'Benefits of growth hormone treatment on bone metabolism, bone density and bone strength in growth hormone deficiency and osteoporosis'. Department of Internal Medicine I-Endocrinology and Metabolism, University Medical Clinic, Heidelberg, Germany. National Library of Medicine, January 15, 2001 http:// www.growthhormonetherapy.cc/

27 Orimo, H. et al. 'Effect of alpha-hydroxyvitamin D3 on lumbar spine bone mineral density and vertebral fractures in patients with postmenopausal osteoporosis'. *Calcified Tissue International* 1994; 54:370–376.

28 Prior, J.C. 'Progesterone as a bone-trophic hormone. *Endocrine Reviews* 1990; 11:386–398.

29 Gaby, A.R. MD. 'Progesterone fails osteoporosis trial', *Townsend Letter* for Doctors and Patients – December 1999, p. 121.

30 Cundy, T. et al. 'Bone density in women receiving depo-medroxyprogesterone acetate for contraception'. *BMJ* 1991; 303:13–16.

31 Lee, J.R. 'Osteoporosis reversal: The role of progesterone'. *International Clinical Nutrition Review* 1990; 10(3):384–391.

32 Leonetti, H.B., Longo, S. and Anasti, J.N. 'Transdermal progesterone cream for

vasomotor symptoms and postmenopausal bone loss'. *Journal of Obstetrics and Gynecology* 1999; 94:225–228.

33 Gaby, A.R. *Preventing and Reversing Osteoporosis*. Prima Health, 1994.

34 Legrain, Sylvie et al. 'Dehydroepiandrosterone replacement administration: pharmacokinetic and pharmacodynamic studies in healthy elderly subjects. *Journal of Clinical Endocrinology and Metabolism* 2000; 85:3208–3217.

35 Alexandersen, P. et al. 'Ipriflavone in the treatment of postmenopausal osteoporosis'. *JAMA* 2000; 285(11):1483–1488.

CHAPTER NINE
The calcium dairy myth

1 Mazess, R.B. 'Bone density in premenopausal women: Effects of age, dietary intake, physical activity, smoking and birth control pills'. *American Journal of Clinical Nutrition* 1991; 53:132–142.

2 Hegsted, D.M. 'Calcium and osteoporosis'. *Journal of Nutrition* 1986; 116:2316–2319.

3 ibid.

4 Anderson, J.B. 'The important role of physical activity in skeletal development: How exercise may counter low calcium intake'. *Am J Clin Nutr* 2000; 71:1384–1386.

5 NIH Consensus Conference. NIH Consensus Development Panel on Optimum Calcium Intake. *JAMA* 1994; 272:1942–1944.
Heaney, R. 'Distribution of calcium absorption in middle-aged women'. *Am J Clin Nutr* 1986; 43:299–305.

6 Dawson-Hughes, B. 'Calcium supplementation and bone loss: A review of clinical trials'. *Am J Clin Nutr* 1991; 54(Suppl.):274–280S.

7 Mazess, R.B. and Barden, H.S. 'Bone density in premenopausal women: Effects of age, dietary intake, physical activity, smoking and birth control pills'. *Am J Clin Nutr* 1991; 53:132–142.

8 Patrick, Lyn. Cited in 'Comparative absorption of calcium sources and calcium citrate malate for the prevention of osteoporosis'. http://www.thorne.com/altmedrev/fulltext/calcium4–2.html

9 Weaver, C. and Plawecki, K. 'Dietary calcium: Adequacy of a vegetarian diet'. *Am J Clin Nutr* 1994; 59(Suppl.):1238–1241S.

10 Wyshak, G. 'Consumption of carbonated drinks by teenage girls associated with bone fractures'. *Archives of Pediatrics and Adolescent Medicine* 2000; 154:542–543, 610–613.

11 Hopper, J.L. and Seeman, E. 'The bone density of female twins

discordant for tobacco use'. *New England Journal of Medicine* 1994; 330:387–392.

12 Nordin, B.E. 'Calcium requirement is a sliding scale'. *Am J Clin Nutr* 2000; 71:1381–1383.

13 Wolf, R.L. et al. 'Factors associated with calcium absorption efficiency in pre and perimenopausal women'. *Am J Clin Nutr* 2000; 72:466–471.

14 Abelow, B.J. et al. 'Cross-cultural association between dietary animal protein and hip fracture: A hypothesis'. *Calcified Tissue International* 1992; 50:14–18.

15 Mazess, R.B. et al. 'Bone density of the spine and femur in adult white females'. *Calcif Tissue Int* August 1999; 65(2):91–99. Sheth, R.D. et al. 'Bone mineral density in geographically diverse adolescent populations'. *Pediatrics* November 1996; 98(5):948–951.

16 Kung, A.W. 'Age-related osteoporosis in Chinese: an evaluation of the response of intestinal calcium absorption and calcitropic hormones to dietary calcium deprivation'. *Am J Clin Nutr* 1998; 68(6):1291–1297.

17 Dibba, B. et al. 'Effect of calcium supplementation on bone mineral accretion in Gambian children accustomed to a low-calcium diet'. *Am J Clin Nutr* 2000; 71(2):544–549. Aspray, T.J. et al.

'Low bone mineral content is common but osteoporotic fractures are rare in elderly rural Gambian women'. *Journal of Bone and Mineral Research* 1996; 11(7):1019–1025.

18 Walker, A. 'Osteoporosis and calcium deficiency', *Am J Clin Nutr* 1965; 16:327–336.

19 Smith, R. 'Epidemiologic studies of osteoporosis in women of Puerto Rico and South-eastern Michigan'. *Clinical Orthopaedics and Related Research* 1966; 45:32.

20 Mazees, R. 'Bone mineral content of North Alaskan Eskimos'. *Am J Clin Nutr* 1974; 27:916–925.

21 Weaver, C.M. 'Dietary calcium: Adequacy of a vegetarian diet'. *Am J Clin Nutr* 1994; 59(Suppl.):1238–1241S.

22 Feskanich, D. et al. 'Milk, dietary calcium and bone fractures in women: A 12-year prospective study'. *American Journal of Public Health* 1997; 87:992–997.

23 Cumming, R. 'Case-control of risk factors for hip fractures in the elderly'. *American Journal of Epidemiology* 1994; 139(5):493–503.

24 Weinsier, R.L. 'Dairy foods and bone health: Examination of the evidence'. *Am J Clin Nutr* 2000; 72:681–689.

25 Press release by New Zealand Dairy Board, November 24 2000.

'Clinically proven Anlene paves the way in bone health'. http://www.newsroom.co.nz/story/33967.html

26 Lau, E.M.C. 'The epidemiology of hip fracture in Asia: An update'. *Osteoporosis International* 1996; Suppl.3:S19–23.

27 Leung, S.F. 'Clinical nutrition in Hong Kong'. *Asia Pacific Journal of Clinical Nutrition* 1993; 2:151–153.

28 Kato, I., Tominaga, S. and Kuroishi, T. 'Relationship between westernisation of dietary habits and mortality from breast and ovarian cancer in Japan'. *Japanese Journal of Cancer Research* 1987; 78:349–357.

29 Plant, Jane. *Your Life in Your Hands*. Virgin Publishing Ltd, 2000, p. 78.

30 Schrezenmeir, J. and Jagla, A. 'Milk and diabetes'. *Journal of the American College of Nutrition* April 2000;19 (Suppl.2):176–190S.

31 Plant, Jane, ibid, p. 89.

32 Rusynyk, R.A, and Still, C.D. 'Lactose intolerance'. *Journal of the American Osteopathic Association* April 2001; 101(Suppl.4.Pt 1):S10–12.

33 Plant, Jane, ibid. p. 91.

34 Plant, Jane, ibid, p. 91.

35 Epstein, Samuel S. 'Unlabeled milk from cows treated with biosynthetic growth hormones: A case of regulatory abdication'.

International Journal of Health Services 1996; 26(1):173–185.

CHAPTER TEN
Dietary and nutritional factors

1 Tucker, K.L. et al. 'Potassium, Magnesium and fruit and vegetable intakes are associated with greater bone mineral density in elderly men and women'. *American Journal of Clinical Nutrition* 1999; 64(4):727–736.

2 Albertazzi, P. et al. 'The effect of dietary soy supplementation on hot flushes'. *Journal of Obstetrics and Gynecology* 1998; 91:6–11.

3 Gallagher, J.C. et al., Creighton University, Omaha. 'The effects of soy isoflavone intake on bone metabolism in postmenopausal women'. Presented to symposium on the role of soy in preventing and treating chronic disease. Brussels, Belgium, 1996.

4 Anderson, J.W. et al. 'Meta-analysis of the effects of soy protein intake on serum lipids'. *New England Journal of Medicine* 1995; 333:276–282. (A meta-analysis of 38 studies.)

5 Ingram, D. et al. 'Case-control study of phytoestrogens and breast cancer'. *The Lancet* 1997; 350:990–994.

6 Aldercreutz, H. 'Phytoestrogens: Epidemiology and a possible role in cancer protection'. *Environmental Health*

Perspectives 1995;
103(Suppl.7):103–112.

7 Murkies, A. 'Phytoestrogens —
what is the current knowledge?'
Australian Family Physician
1998; 27(Suppl.1):S47–51.

8 Kato, I., Tominaga, S. and
Kuroishi, T. 'Relationship
between westernisation of
dietary habits and mortality from
breast and ovarian cancer in
Japan'. *Japanese Journal of
Cancer Research* 1987;
78:349–357.

9 Nagata, C. et al. 'Soy product
consumption seems to protect
against hot flashes'. *American
Journal of Epidemiology* 2001;
153:790–793.

10 Dr Suzanne C. Ho reporting at
the Third Annual Scientific
Meeting of the Hong Kong
Epidemiological Association.
January 2001.

11 Horiuchi, T. et al. 'Effect of soy
protein on bone metabolism in
postmenopausal Japanese
women'. *Osteoporosis
International* 2000; 11(8):
721–724.

12 Potter, S.M., Baum, J.A., Teng,
H. et al. 'Soy protein and
isoflavones: Their effects on
blood lipids and bone density in
postmenopausal women. *Am J
Clin Nutr* 1998;
68(Suppl):1375–1379S.

13 Anderson, J.J.B., Ambrose, W.W.
and Garner, S.C. 'Biphasic effects

of genistein on bone tissue in the
ovariectomized lactating rat
model (44243)'. *Proceedings of
the Society for Experimental
Biology and Medicine* 1998;
217:345–350.

14 Weaver, C.M. 'Dietary calcium:
Adequacy of a vegetarian diet'.
Am J Clin Nutr 1994;
59(Suppl):1238–1241S.

15 Remer, T. and Manz, F.
'Estimation of the renal net acid
excretion by adults consuming
diets containing variable amounts
of protein'. *Am J Clin Nutr* 1994;
59:1356–1361.

16 Sellmeyer, D. et al. 'A high ratio
of dietary animal to vegetable
protein increases the rate of bone
loss and the risk of fracture in
postmenopausal women'. *Am J
Clin Nutr.* 2001; 73:118–122.

17 Feskanich, D. et al. 'Protein
consumption and bone fractures
in women'. *Am J Epidemiol* 1996;
143:472–479.

18 Nordin, B.E.C., Need, A.G.,
Morris, H.A. and Horowitz, M.
'The nature and significance of
the relationship between urinary
sodium and urinary calcium in
women'. *Journal of Nutrition*
1993; 123:1615–1622.

19 Harris, S.S. et al. 'Caffeine and
bone loss in healthy
postmenopausal women'. *Am J
Clin Nutr* 1994; 60:573–578.

20 Lloyd, T. 'Caffeine not linked
to bone loss in postmenopausal

women'. *Journal of the American College of Nutrition* 2000; 19:256–261.

21 From Medscape News May 8, 2001. Garg, R. et al. 'Elderly lack adequate levels of Vitamin D'. Posted at the American Association of Clinical Endocrinologists 10th Annual Meeting, held in San Antonio, Texas.

22 Geinster, J.Y. et al. 'Preliminary report of decreased serum magnesium in postmenopausal osteoporosis'. *Magnesium* 1989; 8:106–109.

23 Stendig-Lindberg, G. et al. 'Trabecular bone density in a two-year controlled trial of peroral magnesium in osteoporosis'. *Magnesium Research* 1993; 6:155–163.

24 Dreosti, I.E. 'Magnesium status and health'. *Nutrition Reviews* 1995; 53(7):S23–27.

25 Dimai, H.P. et al. 'Daily oral magnesium supplementation suppresses bone turnover in young adult males'. *Journal of Clinical Endocrinology and Metabolism* 1998; 83(8):2742–2748.

26 Jones, G. et al. 'Diet in pregnancy linked to bone mineral density in offspring'. *European Journal of Clinical Nutrition* 2000; 54:749–756.

27 Gaby, A. *Preventing and Reversing Osteoporosis*. Prima Health 1994.

28 Gaby, A. ibid.

29 Sojka, J.E. and Weaver, C. 'Magnesium supplementation and osteoporosis'. *Nutrition Reviews* 1995; 53(3):71–80.

30 Heaney, R. and Weaver, C. 'Calcium absorption from kale'. *Am J Clin Nutr* 1990; 51:656–657.

31 *Healthnotes* 2000. www.healthnotes.com

32 Feskanich, D. et al. 'Vitamin K intake and hip fractures in women: A prospective study'. *Am J Clin Nutr* 1999; 69(1):74–79.

33 Booth, S. et al. 'Dietary vitamin K intakes are associated with hip fracture but not with bone mineral density in elderly men and women'. *Am J Clin Nutr* 2000; 71(5):1201–1208.

34 *New Scientist* July 15, 2000:22.

35 Gaby, A. ibid.

36 Gaby, A. ibid.

37 Gaby, A. ibid.

38 Elmstahl, S. et al. 'Increased incidence of fractures in middle-aged and elderly men with low intakes of phosphorus and zinc'. *Osteoporosis International* 1998; 8:333–340.

39 Eaton-Evans, J. et al. 'Copper supplementation and bone mineral density in middle-aged women'. *Proceedings of the Nutrition Society* 1995; 54:191A.

40 *Healthnotes* 2000. ibid.

41 Neilson, F.H. et al. 'Effect of

dietary boron on mineral, estrogen and testosterone metabolism in postmenopausal women'. *Federation of American Societies for Experimental Biology (FASEB)* 1987; 1:394–397.

42 Newnham, R.E. 'The role of boron in human nutrition'. *Journal of Applied Nutrition* 1994; 46:81–85.

43 Eisinger, J. et al. 'Effects of silicon, fluoride, etidronate, and magnesium on bone mineral density: A retrospective study'. *Magnes Res* 1993; 6:247–249.

44 *Healthnotes* 2000. ibid.

45 Hyams, D.E. 'Scurvy, megaloblastic anaemia and osteoporosis'. *British Journal of Clinical Practice* 1963; 17:332–340.

46 Melhus, H. 'Excessive dietary intake of vitamin A is associated with reduced bone mineral density and an increased risk for hip fracture'. *Annals of Internal Medicine* 1998; 129(10):770–778.

47 Seeman, Ego. 'New drugs and new data on old drugs.' 22nd Annual Meeting of the American Society for Bone and Mineral Research. www.medscape.com

48 Kruger, M.C. et al. 'Calcium, gamma-linolenic acid and iecosapentaenoic acid supplementation in senile osteoporosis'. *Aging* 1998; 10:385–394.

CHAPTER ELEVEN
Exercise

1 Calbet, J.A.L. et al. 'High bone mineral density in male élite professional volleyball players'. *Osteoporosis International* 1999; 10:468–474.

2 Wolff, J.J. et al. 'The effect of exercise training programs on bone mass: A meta-analysis of published controlled trials in pre and postmenopausal women'. *Osteoporosis International* 1999; 9:1–12.

3 Bassey, J. 'Osteoporosis and Exercise'. *Bone Alert* 2000; 6:4–6.

4 Robertson, M.C. et al. 'Effectiveness and economic evaluation of a nurse delivered home exercise programme to prevent falls'. 2: A controlled trial in multiple centres. *British Medical Journal* 2001; 322:701–704.

5 Robertson, M.C. et al. ibid.

6 Robertson MC et al. 'Effectiveness and economic evaluation of a nurse delivered home exercise programme to prevent falls'. 1: Randomised controlled trial *BMJ* 2001; 322:697–701.

7 Heinonen, A. 'High-impact exercise and bones of growing girls: A 9-month controlled trial'. *Osteoporosis International* 2000; 11:1010–1017.

8 O'Connor, Deirdre. 'Osteoporosis'. *Alternative*

Medicine Reviews 1997; 2(1):36.
www.thorne.com/altmedrev

9   Lumsden, David B. et al. 'T'ai chi
for osteoarthritis: An introduction
for primary care physicians'.
Geriatrics February 1998;
53:84–88.

10 Wolf, S.L. et al. 'Reducing frailty
and falls in older persons: An
investigation of T'ai Chi and
computerized balance training'.
*Journal of the American
Geriatrics Society* 1996;
44:599–600.

11 TVNZ News. Tuesday May 8,
2001.

12 http://www.meltdown.com/
osteo2.html

13 Chopra, Deepak. *Ageless Body,
Timeless Mind*. p. 86. Random
House 1993.

14 Fiatarone, M.A. 'Exercise
training and nutritional
supplementation for physical
frailty in very elderly people'.
New England Journal of Medicine
1994; 330(25):1769–1775.

15 Christine Gorman. *Time*
magazine February 5, 2000;
157:5.

16 CNN; Science Daily. Reported in
Partners, the AIM magazine. July
1998.

17 O'Connor, Deirdre. ibid.

18 Kerr, D. et al. 'Exercise effects on
bone mass in postmenopausal
women are site-specific and load
dependent'. *Journal of Bone and
Mineral Research* 1996;
11:218–225.

19 Bennell, K. et al. 'The role of
physiotherapy in the prevention
and treatment of osteoporosis'.
Manual Therapy 2000;
5(4):198–213.

20 Bennell, K. et al. ibid.

CONCLUSION

1   Korten, David C. *When
Corporations Rule the World*.
Earthscan Publications 1995:
p. 146.

2   Freidberg, M. et al. 'Evaluation
of conflict of interest in economic
analyses of new drugs used in
oncology'. *Journal of the
American Medical Association*
1999; 282:1453–1457.

3   le Carre, John. 'I'm sickened by
the world of pharmaceuticals'.
The *Vancouver Sun* December
16, 2000.

4   Bassett, Ken. 'On trying to stop
the measurement of bone
density to sell drugs: A tribute to
a friend'. *Tales from Other
Drug Wars*. Papers from the 12th
Annual Health Policy
Conference, held in Vancouver,
B.C. November 26, 1999.
ISBN 0–88865–240–2.

INDEX

231

FURTHER READING

Coney, Sandra, *The Menopause Industry*, Penguin Books (NZ), 1991.

Gaby, Alan R., MD, *Preventing and Reversing Osteoporosis*, Prima Health, 1994.

Nelson, Miriam, *Strong Women, Strong Bones*, Lothian, 1999.

Ott, Susan, MD, 'Osteoporosis and Bone Physiology'.
http://courses.washington.edu/bonephys/opbmd.html#young

Plant, Professor Jane, *Your Life in Your Hands*, Virgin, 2000.

Sanson, Gill, *Mid-Life Energy and Happiness,* Penguin Books (NZ), 1999.

'Bone Mineral Density Testing: Does the evidence support its use in well women?' B.C. Office of Health Technology Assessment. Dec 1997. www.chspr.ubc.ca.

Mundy, Alicia, *Dispensing With The Truth*, St Martin's Press, 2001.